W9-CIG-217

THE NEW SCIENCE
OF FIGHTING
SILENT HEART DISEASE

THE NEW SCIENCE OF FIGHTING SILENT HEART DISEASE

Causes, Diagnoses, Prevention, and Treatments

DR. HAROLD L. KARPMAN, MD

ROWMAN & LITTLEFIELD
Lanham • Boulder • New York • London

Disclaimer: *This book represents reference material only.* It is not intended as a medical manual. This book is not a replacement for treatment(s) that the reader's personal physician may have suggested. If the reader believes he or she is experiencing a medical issue, professional medical help is recommended. Mention of particular products, companies, or authorities in this book does not indicate endorsement by the publisher or author.

Published by Rowman & Littlefield
An imprint of The Rowman & Littlefield Publishing Group, Inc.
4501 Forbes Boulevard, Suite 200, Lanham, Maryland 20706
www.rowman.com

6 Tinworth Street, London SE11 5AL, United Kingdom

Copyright © 2020 by The Rowman & Littlefield Publishing Group, Inc.

All rights reserved. No part of this book may be reproduced in any form or by any electronic or mechanical means, including information storage and retrieval systems, without written permission from the publisher, except by a reviewer who may quote passages in a review.

British Library Cataloguing in Publication Information Available

Library of Congress Cataloging-in-Publication Data

Library of Congress Control Number: 2020939992

ISBN: 978-1-5381-3655-3 (cloth)
ISBN: 978-1-5381-3656-0 (electronic)

To my wife, Molinda, for her encouragement, support, and creative contributions

CONTENTS

INTRODUCTION

Every minute of every day, thousands of people are walking around with the equivalent of a hidden time bomb ticking away in their chests. Silently, painlessly, their hearts are being injured by repeated interruptions of the vital, nourishing flow of blood through the coronary arteries to the heart itself. As time goes by, the heart sustains more and more damage . . . but there is still no pain until the fateful moment when this process all too often reaches its deadly, unexpected conclusion in a massive heart attack or even sudden death.

While scourges like deaths from drug overdoses and Alzheimer's capture the media's and the public's attention, the cold, hard fact of the matter is that heart disease remains the number one killer of American adults—responsible for five times the number of deaths from drug overdoses and Alzheimer's combined. When calculated with the related medical condition known as stroke, cardiovascular disease felled nearly 850,000 U.S. residents in 2017, accounting for one in every three deaths. Cardiovascular disease claims more lives each year than all forms of cancer and chronic respiratory diseases.

About half of all heart attacks are mistaken for less serious problems or completely missed. But make no mistake: "silent" heart attacks can increase your risk of dying from coronary heart disease.

THE ORIGIN STORY OF SILENT HEART DISEASE

Silent myocardial ischemia (SMI), or silent heart disease, is a particularly insidious form of the disease suffered by 25 percent of those with heart conditions. As the name implies, patients suffering from silent heart disease are not aware that their heart is being injured because they feel no pain (or not enough to be concerned). Despite undeniable evidence and decades of research, not to mention new diagnostic tools, the perception by the public and, I'm sorry to say, many members of the medical profession is that unless less there's chest pain (angina), then there's no heart attack or damage to the heart.

In 1970, I broke with the medical orthodoxy of the time that said that unless a heart attack was accompanied by chest pains, it really wasn't a heart attack, and patients and their doctors need not be concerned. My experience as a practicing cardiologist, the cofounder of a cardiology practice in Beverly Hills, California, and a clinical professor at UCLA's school of medicine told me otherwise.

Two years earlier, my two partners, Drs. Daniel and Selvyn Bleifer, and I had purchased an early diagnostic machine, the Holter electrocardiograph, which used magnetic tape to record electrical cardio impulses through the human body. It weighed eighty-five pounds, but it was state of the art at the time and, most importantly, ushered in a whole new dimension in cardiology. Instead of just examining the heart with the standard electrocardiogram for a period of one minute—hardly adequate for a comprehensive evaluation—the Holter equipment permitted evaluation of up to twenty-four hours of heart action. The patient's heart now could be studied in the patient's home or office, not just in the doctor's examination room or medical lab. It was the precursor to today's wearable health devices.

We could now evaluate the effects of stress or ordinary living and working activities on heart action and coronary artery blood flow. Getting this information was vitally important since 95 percent of all heart attacks are caused by restriction of blood flow in the heart's arteries, typically caused by the buildup of plaque or various substances, notably the waxy, organic stuff called cholesterol.

Based on our new research using the new and improved diagnostics, as well as our own clinical observation over twenty years, we were pretty sure that the old trope that a heart attack must be accompanied by chest pain (otherwise, it was not a heart attack) was dead wrong. In September 1970, we presented our research findings at the Sixth World Congress of Cardiology in London, attended by thousands of the world's leading heart doctors. In a paper titled "Clinical Applications of Dynamic Electrocardiography," we proved conclusively that our suspected silent heart disease was in fact a real condition likely suffered by tens of millions of unknowing adults worldwide.

Then we waited for the accolades to pour in for what was obviously our groundbreaking work. They didn't. The reaction among the cardiology profession was more a trickle of acknowledgment than a tidal wave of acceptance.

As it turns out, most physicians were wholly unfamiliar with the development of the then modern-day diagnostic equipment, since the Holter had been in use for only two to three years before the conference and in widely scattered medical facilities at that. For the average physician attending the event, we might as well have been saying that our friends on Mars had beamed the information to us. To be clear, relatively few cardiologists were convinced the newfangled electrocardiograph equipment was significant, and still fewer believed in our hypothesized silent heart disease.

Essentially, the "no pain, no heart attack" school won the day. The battle, yes, but not the war.

Over the next seven years, the Holter and other electrocardiographic recording devices became more prevalent and more sophisticated. Additional studies by Drs. Daniel Tzivone and Shlomo Stern in Israel in 1974 suggested these painless episodes of poor coronary artery blood flow could occur even during resting activities—another heresy, since it was widely believed that strenuous activity was usually a precursor to a heart attack. Imagine, then, if significant and even life-threatening heart damage was occurring all the time while patients were relaxing and with no indication of any chest pain. Impossible!

However, year after year additional studies confirmed our earlier research, including one in 1977 by Drs. Steven Schange and Carl Pepine from the University of Florida, which confirmed that as many as four episodes of silent heart disease occur for every episode of chest pain. You see, it was not an either/or proposition—angina or silent ischemia—but oftentimes both.

By 1983, the tide was beginning to turn as more studies using other kinds of rapidly developing diagnostic techniques, such as treadmill testing, radioactive isotopes, and echocardiography, confirmed the widespread existence of silent heart disease. The benchmark symptom of chest pain as the exclusive indicator of heart damage was crumbling before the facts.

In 1989, I compiled my own research as well as subsequent medical studies into the first book ever written on the topic for the consumer, *Preventing Silent Heart Disease: Detecting and Preventing America's Number 1 Killer*. Now, three decades later, I have written this entirely new book, *The New Science of Fighting Silent Heart Disease*. In brief, the book shows the average reader what to do and how to do it to reduce the chances of developing or even to reverse the effects of silent heart disease.

Much has changed and much has remained the same over the thirty years since I wrote the first book. Heart disease remains the nation's number one killer of men and women. However, today new technologies and science for detecting, treating, and preventing coronary disease and its most insidious manifestation—silent heart disease and sudden death—can empower virtually everyone to take the necessary steps to avoid falling victim to the silent killer.

HOW TO USE THIS BOOK

Let's do a quick recap: On average, 45 percent of all heart attacks are silent—that is, they are painless and leave behind damage that remains undetected, unless the patient and his or her doctor are looking for it. Silent heart disease is the main cause of sudden death; it is American's number one public health problem, with more than six hundred thousand sudden deaths and 1.5 million heart attacks occurring in the United States each year. This book tells you what you need to know in order to vanquish this silent killer.

The book is divided into four parts. Part I provides background on how the heart works and what happens when it doesn't. It's important to know the basic biology of the heart muscle and coronary artery disease to fully understand silent heart disease.

Part II provides an overview of what we know today about the causes of silent heart disease since my colleagues and I first identified the condition in the 1970s. Today we know the disease is the result of both inherited and environmental causes—a combination of nature and nurture somewhat unique to each individual. We look into the leading risk factors and how they've changed—in some instances, quite dramatically for the worse. The idea here is not to scare but to inform; knowledge is power. The better we understand the risk factors for and mechanisms of silent heart disease, the more effective we can be in fighting it.

In Part III, we discuss the best in detection and treatment techniques proven over the last five decades, as well as the latest in diagnostic tools, new medications, recent surgical innovations, and cutting-edge treatments, from gene therapy and stem cell manipulation to bioprinting and implantable devices. As someone on the frontlines of fighting silent heart disease for the better half of a century, I can say that many of today's treatments would have been considered science fiction just a generation ago, and even more fantastic innovations are on the near horizon.

In Parts II and III you'll also encounter case studies taken from my medical practice files, which will illustrate key points. They're all based on real-life patients of mine; only their names have been changed to protect their privacy.

In Part IV, the final part of the book, you become part of the solution. By taking an easy, self-administered test, you determine your "risk profile." A necessary word of caution: Always consult with your physician before proceeding with any changes in your health regimen. The information provided in this book is meant to educate, not instruct.

Now, let's get started on our journey to preventing silent heart disease.

Part I

ANATOMY OF A SILENT KILLER

PART I: INTRODUCTION

You would know if you had a heart attack, right? Movies and TV shows are filled with depictions of people in the throes of the gripping chest pain of a heart attack, or myocardial infarction (in medical parlance). But here's the thing: nearly one in two people who experience a heart attack are unaware they're having one.

A silent myocardial ischemia (SMI), or silent heart attack for the purposes of this book, affects 45 percent, or nearly half, of all heart attack victims, according to the most comprehensive study to date. The Atherosclerosis Risk in Communities (ARIC) Study tracked 9,498 participants of different genders and races, with ages ranging from the forties to the eighties, over a span of a decade. This kind of study, with its longevity—ten years—and its use of real-life people in everyday circumstances, is, by the way, the gold standard for scientific medical research versus the typical study using lab mice over the course of a few months.

Until recently, the accepted estimate of silent or painless heart attacks, a manifestation of silent heart disease, as a portion of total heart attacks was thought to have been only 25 percent, so the latest research nearly doubles the risk that Americans face from silent heart disease. Let's do the numbers: more than a million Americans have heart attacks every year, and nearly half of them have no idea of the damage being done.

Part of the reason so many Americans suffer from heart disease in general and silent heart disease in particular is because they lack a basic understanding of heart function and dysfunction. Remember that the mantra for this book is knowledge is power; the more you know about your heart, the more empowered you will be as a patient. So consider the four chapters in Part I of this book your heart-health primer. Now, it may remind you a bit of school homework, but the difference is that everybody gets an A for just reading it.

1

HEART BIOLOGY 101

There's a reason artificial hearts have been, at best, a grand experiment (although 3-D bioprinting offers intriguing possibilities, as we'll explore in Part III). Simply put, the human heart is a magnificent biological machine, at once exceedingly complex and elegantly simple.

If all the blood vessels in the human body, big and small, were laid end to end, the resulting tube would be an incredible 12,400 miles long. Every diagnostic and therapeutic tool in the field of cardiology is dedicated to preserving the ability of the heart to function efficiently as the main element of a simple system, which effectively pumps blood through this long tube. This is the heart's only purpose; it has no other role.

So let's take a quick journey along this 12,400-mile pathway to see exactly how your heart works.

The heart is a hollow, muscular, four-chambered organ that is about the size of an adult fist and weighs less than one pound. It lies slightly to the left of the middle of the chest and is protected by the breastbone and the ribs. The major pumping chamber of the heart, the left ventricle, is a thick-walled compartment that delivers blood into one end of the long vascular tube with sufficient pressure to pump the fluid along its entire length. After the oxygen and nutrients carried in the blood have been removed by the various organs and tissues located along the length of the arterial system, the blood is returned at extremely low pressure, via the venous system, to the right atrium, the lower collecting chamber on the right side of the heart.

It next goes through the tricuspid valve to the relatively thin-walled right ventricle, which then gently ejects the blood still under relatively low pressure across the pulmonic valve into the lungs. The 300 million air sacs located in the lungs enrich the blood with oxygen obtained from the air we breathe. Simultaneously, carbon dioxide gas is removed from the blood and exhaled into the air. The oxygen-enriched blood then moves, still under relatively low pressure, into the lower collecting chamber of the left side of the heart, the left atrium.

It next goes through the well-known mitral valve (the one that is frequently affected in patients with rheumatic heart disease) into the workhorse of the heart, the lower left chamber, called the left ventricle. The internal pressure in the left ventricle increases dramatically, and then, approximately once each second, this extremely strong and efficient chamber ejects the blood forcefully out of the heart through the aortic valve into the aorta, the body's main artery.

The right and left coronary arteries branch off the aorta at its very beginning, and they then divide first into a few major arteries, next into many medium-sized arteries, and finally into thousands of smaller and smaller arteries, which transport the blood to every part of the body.

Each of the smallest blood vessels (called arterioles) gives rise to a network of even smaller blood-carrying tubules known as capillaries, which reach out to nourish the tiny tissue cells themselves. The thin walls of the capillaries permit oxygen and nutrients to be absorbed by the cells and tissues and, in turn, receive waste products, which are first carried back to the heart by the venous system and then transported to the lungs and kidneys by the arterial system for proper disposal.

AN INCREDIBLE PUMP!

The four heart valves (aortic, pulmonic, mitral, and tricuspid) normally allow blood to flow in only one direction, without backflow or leakage. (When leakage does occur as a result of injury or disease—for example, due to rheumatic heart disease or infection—the efficiency of the heart as a pump becomes impaired and permanent damage may result.) The blood simply circulates like water in a fountain with a closed circuit. The water is pumped out the top of the fountain, flows to the bottom, and then is pumped under high pressure to spray once again out the top. It all sounds a bit complicated but is really quite simple.

And what an incredible pump it is! No mechanical pump of equal capacity has been devised by humans with similar efficiency, longevity, and reliability. Consider the following facts: The normal heart beats between 87,000 and 144,000 times per day. During the average lifetime, the heart will beat over 2.5 billion times, moving well over 50 million gallons of blood. The two thousand gallons of blood pumped daily are fully recirculated every ten to fifteen seconds.

The heart is like all other organs—it too must receive fresh oxygenated blood filled with life-giving nutrients if it is to survive and continue its vigorous pumping activities. The coronary arteries comprise the superb personal circulatory system, which nourishes this miraculous pump. (The word "coronary" is derived from the Latin word *corona*, meaning "crown," as in a king's crown, which pictorially describes the arrangement of these arteries on the surface of the heart.)

The coronary arteries are the very first that branch off the aorta as it receives blood from the left ventricle. The all-important left coronary artery nourishes most of the left ventricle, and the right coronary artery carries blood to the walls of the right ventricle as well as to the back and lower surfaces of the heart.

Tiny terminal branches called collateral arteries connect the circulation between the two sides. These connecting arteries are called into play when the circulation to one side of the heart or the other is diminished. When this occurs, fresh blood can still reach the region of the heart deprived of its usual blood flow through this physiological "back door." This backup system tends to enlarge for the several weeks after a coronary artery is obstructed, and it can even grow large enough to prevent another heart attack if a second coronary artery later becomes blocked.

The right coronary artery divides into smaller arteries at a relatively distant location along its path; the left coronary artery, however, quickly splits into two major branches, the left anterior descending and the left circumflex arteries. "Triple vessel disease" describes patients afflicted with severe narrowing or blockage of three coronary arteries, usually the left anterior descending, the left circumflex, and the right coronary arteries. When a patient requires five or six grafts during a coronary artery bypass operation, the grafts will usually include replacements for these three vessels as well as two or three of their branches.

BATTERIES AND WIRES

The heart is a model of efficiency and uniformity; its regularity is due to tiny electric impulses that are self-generated on an average of once every second by the sinoatrial node, the natural electrical "battery" pacemaker of the heart. This tiny "battery" automatically generates electric currents, which are conducted along a system of "wires" within the heart muscle itself. If the sinoatrial node fails to operate properly, its function is taken up by one of a series of backup "batteries" scattered throughout the heart. They usually are activated only when the heart's primary pacemaker fails or if a malfunction occurs in its electrical conduction system.

The pumping chambers are sparked in a carefully timed sequence by the currents generated in the sinoatrial node; the net result is a contraction or squeezing down of these chambers in an orderly fashion, at the appropriate time. The blood is forced to systematically flow from the upper chambers (the atria) to the lower chambers (the ventricles) and then into the general circulation—specifically, to the lungs from the right ventricle and to the rest of the body from the left ventricle. This harmonious efficiency would be destroyed if a malfunction were to occur in one or more of the three major regions described above: (1) in the sinoatrial node (the "battery"), (2) in the conducting "wires," or (3) in the "pump" (heart muscle) itself.

BUILT-IN REDUNDANCY

Oxygenated blood is pumped from the left ventricle into the coronary arteries, which carry the blood over the heart's surface to its most distant regions and then penetrate the heart muscle itself. These indispensable supply lines provide nutrition for all parts of this incredible pumping organ, which normally operates with harmonious efficiency. However, if the blood flow through to the arteries becomes inadequate due to atherosclerotic injury or narrowing, the heart's perfect timing can be affected, likely because of resulting damage to one of its component parts (battery, wires, pump), thereby diminishing or destroying the heart's ability to nourish the various organs of the body, including itself.

Nature has been kind to us in many ways. For example, we have two eyes, two kidneys, and two adrenal glands. If we lose one, we always have the other to take up the function of its lost partner, and it usually does so quite successfully. It's nature's grand plan for built-in redundancy. If system one fails, then switch to its identical twin system. It's a concept embraced by mechanical engineering, architecture, aeronautics . . . any system that has unacceptable consequences if the primary system fails.

Even though we have only one heart, nature has again thoughtfully provided a backup feature, an enormous safety factor. If a significant portion of the heart is lost due to damage or injury, temporary or permanent, the remaining portion of the heart will usually take on the load and carry on quite nicely, albeit somewhat less efficiently. A heart that has been permanently damaged due to a heart attack will frequently last as long and be almost as efficient as a healthy heart, unless the damage is extremely large or critically placed. In fact, one can usually get along quite well for many years (or even for a normal life span) if only 5 or 10 percent of the heart has been damaged.

If the degree of damage is very severe, physical incapacity may result, and frequently the life span will be shortened. Therefore, we do everything we can to preserve the heart, to prevent damage, and, if damage does occur, to limit the size of the injury. The contemporary approach to treatment of an acute heart attack is aggressively dedicated to the prevention of complications and to saving as much heart muscle as is possible.

2

WHY DO HEART ATTACKS HAPPEN?

I know what you're thinking. I've just extolled the virtues of that magnificent biological pumping machine (with built-in redundancy) that we call the human heart. So why are there so many heart attacks? According to the latest figures from the Centers for Disease Control (CDC), approximately 1.5 million heart attacks and related strokes occur every year in the United States, and more than eight hundred thousand people die each year from a "failed heart" caused by cardiovascular disease.

That's a lot of heart problems.

So, why does it happen? The short answer is that there are many reasons why heart attacks happen. Practically speaking, however, the vast majority of heart attacks have one simple cause: not enough blood is flowing through one or more of the coronary arteries. In most instances, the flow is blocked by fatty deposits in the coronary arteries that build up at an extremely slow rate, thickening and hardening the arteries, causing atherosclerosis (or arteriosclerosis). The accumulation of this porridge-like material first narrows and then eventually may completely block the coronary arteries.

A heart attack occurs, as a rule, only when the artery becomes completely blocked. But it has become quite clear in recent years that major problems can arise even when the arteries are only minimally or moderately narrowed by the atherosclerosis. Oxygen starvation of the heart is the most important cause of angina (chest pain), the death of heart tissue ("heart attacks"), malfunctions of heart rhythms (palpitations or "skipping" of the heart), and sudden death.

Completely silent (painless) episodes of heart oxygen starvation may occur anytime, even at the beginning of the atherosclerotic process, when the fatty material is just beginning to be deposited in the coronary arteries and even though significant blockages have not yet developed.

Silent heart attacks are by definition painless or at least free of the classic symptom (a gripping pain in the chest). The undetected transient or momentary decrease of coronary artery blood supply that causes a silent heart attack may last for only a few seconds or, on the other hand, for many minutes or even hours.

RETHINKING HEART EVENTS

For obvious reasons, cardiologists and pathologists in past years have focused only on atherosclerotic blockage of the coronary arteries as the principle cause of heart attacks, malfunctions of heart rhythms, and/ or sudden death. In fact, obstruction of the blood flow in the coronary arteries by atherosclerotic fatty deposits was, and still is, considered to be the single most important cause of these events. But scientific evidence is forcing doctors to go beyond the concept of simple narrowing or blockage of a coronary artery to that of a more dynamic and complex process being responsible for most coronary heart problems.

Both silent and painful coronary heart problems are caused by narrowing or complete blockage of the coronary arteries resulting from various permutations and combinations of intermittently active narrowing of the muscular coronary artery wall in regions of fixed arteriosclerotic plaque. In other words, if the lumen (passageway) of a coronary artery has been narrowed to, say, 70 percent of its normal size by a cholesterol plaque, it may be yet further narrowed (or completely closed) by spasm of the arterial wall itself or by an unpredictable and intermittently increased tendency for rapidly flowing blood to clot in certain key locations in the heart chamber or in the coronary arteries.

Episodes of poor coronary artery blood flow, or ischemia, in silent heart disease, are totally symptom-free (no pain or other warning sensations) in at least three out of four instances. In virtually all cases the telltale signs of a painless heart strain or attack are detectable even in these very early stages with relatively simple tests.

I'm reminded of a patient of mine—a famous Hollywood actress— who was convinced that she was not a candidate for silent heart disease, even though she had several risk factors that indicated otherwise. I knew her socially, so finally after much cajoling, I convinced her to visit my office at the Southern California Cardiology Group in Beverly Hills. By the time her exam was over, it was clear she was suffering from silent heart disease and had already had several silent (painless) heart attacks. She was on the verge of a massive, and potentially fatal, heart attack. When I showed her the results of her diagnostic tests, she could hardly believe her eyes, but at last she was convinced of the danger. She immediately embraced a treatment regimen specific to her medical condition and risk factors. I'm happy to report that she continues today to pursue an active career in film and television.

The point here is that early discovery of ischemia, especially in the symptom-free individual, is terribly important since the person may never know that she or he is afflicted with heart disease until an acute heart attack or failure. In fact, sudden death may be the first sign of a heart problem in many unfortunate cases. Because physicians in the past have relied primarily upon angina (chest pain) to alert them to the onset of significant coronary heart disease, the true onset of meaningful heart disease has frequently not been detected during the smoldering days, weeks, or years prior to the onset of symptoms or the occurrence of sudden death.

THE JIM FIXX PHENOMENON

When Jim Fixx first took up running, he was an overweight magazine editor who smoked two packs of cigarettes a day. In the first race he ever ran, when he was thirty-five years old, he came in last in a field of fifty runners with a sixty-year-old man handily beating him. Still, he famously did not give up and went on to write a book that helped to launch the fitness boom in the 1970s, *The Complete Book of Running*. The book remained on the *New York Times* best-seller list for two years and made him a millionaire.

The book became a bible for joggers everywhere because Fixx preached a gospel that was compelling: virtually anyone can run (you don't need special training or equipment), and running will make you healthier. Those arguments were, well, hard to argue with. There's no doubt that aerobic exercise like running does make you healthier for a variety of reasons.

The great irony of James Fixx's life was his death: he died of a massive heart attack caused by silent heart disease while on a solitary jog in Vermont at the age of fifty-two. How a man who was the picture of perfect health died so suddenly and unexpectedly had to do with how the heart works.

The amount of blood ejected from the heart at any time depends on the body's needs at that moment. More blood is required if one is exercising, experiencing anxiety or stress, or taking certain drugs. These activities cause the heart to beat faster. Thus, the heart itself requires more blood to be delivered through the coronary arteries to nourish the heart muscle.

The amount of blood being delivered through abnormally narrowed or diseased arteries may be more than adequate to supply the needs of a heart beating at a slow or resting rate if the body's requirements are relatively minimal, such as when sleeping or resting. But if the body's blood-flow requirements are increased—for example, with exercise—the heart rate speeds up, and there is a resulting need for more blood flow through the coronary arteries.

If this demand for increased blood flow is beyond the ability of the narrowed arteries to deliver, a significant heart reaction or event, notably chest pain or a heart attack, will occur. Surprisingly enough, most episodes of ischemia in patients with and without angina pectoris (chest pain) are not brought on by increases in the heart rate. Only rarely does the heart rate increase, usually at the very beginning of a period of ischemia.

In the case of James Fixx, his autopsy revealed that two of his coronary arteries were sufficiently blocked to have warranted a bypass operation. According to his friends and family, he had no physical warning signs of heart disease (no pain), although he had a family history of heart disease and was a former smoker.

Unfortunately, the premature and, yes, ironic death of Jim Fixx reinforced a popular misconception: too much exercise will kill you.

In fact, the heart rate associated with most episodes of silent heart disease is usually significantly lower than the rates observed in the same patient while on a treadmill (even when the heart rate is much higher because of the effects of exercise). Silent heart disease frequently occurs in patients with only minimally narrowed, fixed arteriosclerotic lesions (when the artery is narrowed only by 20 to 30 percent).

This symptom-free transient coronary artery narrowing or blockage is caused by a sudden artery spasm. Spasm in the coronary circulation is particularly ominous, since it usually occurs quite suddenly and without warning, in diseased or even in perfectly normal arteries, commonly when the heart rate is slow or normal. Thus, a silent heart disease episode may not be triggered by a stress test (treadmill test) and may therefore not be detected.

Episodes of silent heart disease are probably due to transient decreases in coronary artery blood flow rather than simply due to increases in oxygen need precipitated by the increased heart rates produced by exercise, emotions, drugs, and so forth. A combination of these factors is almost certainly present in every patient with silent heart disease. The concept of chest pain caused by a fast heart rate as the only warning sign of heart disease is no longer accepted by the medical profession. We now know most episodes of inadequate blood flow to the heart are not painful and are not caused or triggered by an increased heart rate.

As it turns out, Jim Fixx likely suffered at least some of his fatal coronary damage from his silent heart disease when he was watching television at night as opposed to when he was vigorously training for his next race.

IT'S NIGHT AND DAY

The sequence of occurrence, magnitude, and duration of episodes of silent heart disease are totally unpredictable for the individual patient, but certain key patterns have emerged over the past three decades. Episodes can occur in the same patient with angina (chest pain) on one occasion and without angina on another. Such episodes may be prolonged at some times and quite brief at others.

It is interesting to note that chest pain may develop toward the end of episodes of myocardial ischemia (partial or complete blockage of a coronary artery), which in the beginning are virtually silent. It's not an either-or proposition—either no pain or intense chest pain—as many patients experience both. Even in those patients who do not have chest pain, considerable overlap may exist between silent and painful episodes. Ischemia (inadequate blood supply) may be present for sixty minutes or longer or may be as brief as 10 to 15 seconds.

In 1983, Drs. John Deanfield, Andrew Selwyn, and their colleagues in London clearly demonstrated that the greatest frequency of both painful and pain-free episodes took place in the morning between 6:00 a.m. and 12 p.m. When this data was analyzed for "time of awakening," the early-morning increase of silent heart disease episodes was striking. More episodes took place in the first and second hour after patients rose, at a time when they were least likely to be exerting themselves and their heart rates were usually quite slow. The episodes were found to generally follow a twenty-four-hour, biological time sequence known as the circadian rhythm pattern.

Subsequent research over the past thirty years has reconfirmed the finding that our circadian clocks are tightly related to cardiovascular functions. New research has shown a strong correlation between disruption of circadian rhythms and cardiovascular events like heart attacks. As we'll learn in Part II, disruptive sleep patterns including sleep apnea are a significant risk factor for silent heart disease. Given the disruptions to normal circadian rhythms caused by life in the modern world—shift work, artificial light, transmeridian air flight, and smartphones—you see why cardiologists are concerned by silent heart disease risk factors that did not even exist a couple of generations ago.

Heart attacks have been found to be randomly distributed throughout the months of the year and the days of the week; their onsets tend to follow the same circadian pattern as do episodes of silent heart disease, occurring more frequently from 6 a.m. to 12 p.m., with the maximum number between 9 a.m. and 10 a.m.

It is interesting to note that these findings are consistent across all classifications of patients, old and young, men and women, smokers and nonsmokers, coffee drinkers and non–coffee drinkers. It doesn't even matter if the patient has had a previous history of angina (chest pain) or heart attack; the pattern is the same in this case as for those who have no such history.

BLOOD CLOTS AND STRESS HORMONES

We know that approximately 90 percent of all heart attacks are caused by an arteriosclerotic nodule or plaque mostly made up of cholesterol and frequently found to be ruptured or spontaneously broken up, resulting in blockage of a coronary artery. It should be clear, however, that heart attacks occur not simply because of the plaque rupture itself but also because of the enlargement of the blood thrombus (or clot) that forms around the plaque (usually following rupture) and blocks the flow of blood through a coronary artery.

Clotting occurs because there is the tendency for blood elements known as platelets to clump together, quite possibly because of an increased production of the "stress hormones" adrenalin and noradrenaline (i.e., epinephrine and norepinephrine) by one of the body's special nervous systems, the sympathetic nervous system. Other factors may also be important in facilitating blood clotting, but platelet clumping appears to be the main cause. Simple aspirin is still one of the best drugs we have to prevent platelet clumping, and it is widely used to prevent and treat heart attacks. For a while studies indicated that virtually all adults could benefit from taking a children's dosage of aspirin every day; however, subsequent research showed that this isn't the case. The only true beneficiaries of a daily aspirin regimen are those who have previously had a heart event or are at risk of heart disease (again, for a variety of factors that we will explore later in the book).

While plaque rupture and associated blood clotting are considered to be the most important trigger mechanisms of heart attacks, a host of other physiological mechanisms may also occur, usually in the early morning hours. First, there is frequently a blood pressure surge of twenty to thirty millimeters of mercury, which increases the likelihood of plaque rupture. Next, the muscular tension in the walls of the coronary arteries may increase, and if this transient increase in muscle tone is superimposed on a previously existing critical narrowing of the artery, further narrowing, decreased blood flow, and predisposition toward a complete blockage of the artery may occur.

A combination of these events and possibly others appears to be responsible for the clear-cut fact that heart attacks, with or without pain, and sudden death tend to occur more frequently during the morning hours. This information has proven to be of extraordinary value in designing a preventative program to avoid these events. Coronary artery spasm severe enough to cause an acute heart attack or sudden death is a complex and dynamic process that may occur even when the fixed arteriosclerotic narrowing in a coronary artery is relatively minor. These events may happen especially if, at the very moment of artery spasm, there is an increased demand for more coronary artery blood flow because of a rapid heart rate in response to exercise, stress, and/or drugs. A dynamic response such as constriction (and therefore narrowing) of a coronary artery occurs in seconds, thrombosis or clotting occurs in minutes, and development of atherosclerotic lesions requires many months or years.

The overall process starts when we are extremely young and ends with the heart damaged or even death of the heart. So, if narrowing of the arteries is the main culprit in ischemic heart disease, the question becomes, What causes clogged arteries? In other words, why do arteries become clogged with cholesterol plaques? That is precisely the question we'll be tackling in Part II. But until then, it's time for a closer look at the types of silent heart disease in Chapter 3 and ways the heart can become permanently damaged in Chapter 4.

3

TYPES OF SILENT HEART DISEASE

Silent heart disease is usually the result of an inadequate supply of coronary artery blood—and here comes the important part—that is pain-free. It's "silent" because it gives no clues, such as chest pain, that suggests strain or damage to the heart. Within that narrow definition of silent heart disease, there are variations.

In April 1986, a group of prominent cardiologists met at the request of the National Heart Institute in Bethesda, Maryland. They defined silent myocardial ischemia—what we're referring to in this book as silent heart disease—and devised a classification system. Symptom-free patients without a history of heart disease but afflicted with intermittently inadequate coronary artery blood flow were henceforth to be called Type 1; those with symptom-free silent heart disease who had previously suffered a heart attack would be called Type 2; and patients afflicted with or without anginal chest pains and constricted arteries who had not previously suffered a heart attack would be Type 3.

This categorization was more than an academic exercise because with each silent heart disease classification came a singular set of challenges.

TYPE 1 (COMPLETELY SILENT)

If silent heart disease is diagnosed in a symptom-free patient, the outlook is as grave as it is for a similar patient with angina pains; in other words, silent heart disease is bad whether it is associated with chest pain or not.

TYPE 2 (WITH HEART ATTACK HISTORY)

Contrary to popular belief, most people today do not die from a heart attack. In fact, 90 percent survive. That wasn't the case just a few decades ago when nearly half of heart attack victims died within a few days.

The survivors of heart attacks living in the United States form an extremely large, growing, and readily identifiable subset of patients with known coronary heart disease. This group in aggregate now totals at least 5 million. It's no small irony that while the death rate due to heart disease among the general population has decreased over the last twenty years, the rate of those who suffer from heart disease has increased because good medical therapy has increased the number of heart attack survivors.

Over the past decade, it has become common practice to perform a low-level stress test on heart attack subjects one to three weeks after the acute heart injury has occurred. The cardiologist uses this test to be assured that patients are able to resume the increasingly vigorous physical activities required of them when they return home from the hospital without developing signs or symptoms suggestive of heart ischemia or rhythm malfunctions. Routine and/or thallium stress testing is also extensively employed weeks, months, and years after a heart attack in order to determine (1) the functional capacity of the heart, including its ability to withstand an increased heart rate such as might occur in stressful or even relatively ordinary activities, and (2) whether or not silent heart disease is present.

It has been estimated that at least 40 percent of the 1 million heart attack survivors in the United States each year will subsequently have abnormal treadmill stress tests, with 50 percent of these having been symptom-free—the classic Type 2 patient. Similarly, wearable monitoring devices reveal that that as many as 33 percent of heart attack survivors will have silent heart disease.

Post–heart attack patients who demonstrate pain-free ischemia on either test have a much higher incidence of recurrent heart attacks, new onset of anginal chest pain, and sudden death than do patients who do not demonstrate changes on these tests.

To frame it another way, patients afflicted with silent heart disease after a heart attack are ten times more likely to die within one year than are patients without symptoms, and almost one-third of them do. Finding silent heart disease in these patients is important because it can be treated, and the incidence of serious health problems and death thus can be reduced or eliminated.

TYPE 3 (WITH CHEST PAIN)

The millions of Americans who have silent heart disease and angina are more likely to have an early adverse outcome, including recurrent heart attacks, increasing angina, or even sudden death, than are the angina patients without silent heart disease. Wait a minute, you're probably thinking. Didn't we earlier define silent heart disease as symptom-free, painless ischemia (inadequate blood flow to the heart)? Can a patient have it both ways?

The answer is yes. Some patients do have it both ways—inadequate blood flow to the heart, sometimes with pain and at other times without pain; sometimes the condition is symptomatic and at other times asymptomatic. We know this because patients might experience chest pains for the first time and go to a cardiologist, who confirms their chest pains are symptomatic of an intermittently constricted blood flow to the heart. But guess what? Further diagnostic analysis shows the telltale damage to the heart was caused by past, painless episodes of silent heart disease or classic angina pectoris resulting in heart scars.

It is of utmost importance to properly and carefully study all angina patients with exercise testing and/or Holter recording (more on this later) to determine if silent ischemia is present. Research indicates that EKG abnormalities on treadmill or Holter tests may even occur more frequently in patients without chest pain than in patients with chest pain.

THE IMPORTANCE OF CHEST PAIN

The outlook for developing cardiac complications or sudden death is related to the presence and degree of inadequate blood flow to the heart, painful or not.

Ironically, chest pain can be a life-saving warning if addressed in time. Symptom-free, high-risk heart patients with numerous risk factors (smoking, high cholesterol, high blood pressure, positive family history, all of which we'll explore in Part 2) have a much higher mortality rate from heart attacks and incidence of sudden death than do patients without abnormal risk factors, angina, and/or known coronary heart disease. Patients with silent heart disease who have previously suffered an acute heart attack or who have unstable angina are at very high risk for death and recurrent heart attacks compared to similar patients without silent heart disease and/or a history of cardiac symptoms or events. Diabetics and high-blood-pressure patients are particularly prone to silent heart disease and silent (symptom-free) heart attacks.

The absence of pain does not mean that silent heart disease is benign. Although approximately 50 percent of all patients with significant heart disease go to their physicians because of chest pain or other symptoms, sudden death or an acute heart attack is the initial event for the other 50 percent. The vast majority of patients with symptom-free heart disease do not seek medical attention because they are totally unaware of their life-threatening heart condition.

It is imperative that doctors identify which patients have symptom-free heart disease, because we now have specific therapies available that can delay or possibly even prevent heart attacks or sudden death. Let's remind ourselves one more time: physicians and patients should not rely on chest pains as the first warning of a significant heart condition.

UNSTABLE ANGINA

While we refer to the classic heart attack as being characterized by chest pain, it's more than that. Angina pectoris literally means "choking in the chest," and the pain experienced by patients suffering from it is unique. Some describe it as a heaviness on the chest, others as an extreme tightness or squeezing, often accompanied by extreme fatigue.

The association between heart attack and angina is literally engrained in medical history, which why it was initially so difficult for my colleagues and me, over thirty years, to convince our fellow cardiologists that there was such a thing as silent heart disease.

No doubt, the ancients experienced heart disease and heart attacks. We know that because modern-day diagnostic technology has revealed the signs of it in Egyptian mummies. The Romans, who were fanatical about recording everyday life, mention symptoms associated with heart attack and heart disease but made no connection between the symptoms and the pathology of heart disease.

Likely the first written account of heart disease was by a seventh-century Arab poet who was lovesick, mourning for a partner forced to marry another and move away:

> My heart is firmly seized
> By a bird's claws;
> My heart is tightly squeezed,
> When Lila's name flows.
> My body is tightly bound,
> My body is tightly bound,
> Is like a finger ring around.

That certainly sounds like angina to me, and indeed, as we'll learn later, stress hormones caused by extreme emotional anxiety can facilitate a heart event that is colloquially called a "broken heart."

Renaissance man Leonardo da Vinci (1452–1519) was the first to investigate and then record his finding of pathology in the coronary arteries. William Harvey (1578–1657), King Charles I of England's personal royal physician, discovered that blood moves around the body in a circulatory manner from the heart, an important next step in understanding the connection between angina and heart attack. German professor of medicine Friedrich Hoffmann (1660–1742), in his classic medical text, observed that coronary heart disease started in the areas where there is a "reduced passage of the blood within the coronary arteries." Credit Americans William Osler (1849–1919) and James B. Herrick (1861–1954) for the determination that the narrowing of the coronary arteries was the most likely cause of angina and heart attacks.

When angina is of new onset, when it suddenly increases in intensity, frequency, or duration, and happens repeatedly, occurring even at rest or with only minimal exertion, or when it is associated with profuse sweating, nausea, vomiting, shortness of breath, rapid palpitations, or profound malaise, it is called unstable angina. This is a sign of an impending or evolving acute heart attack. It is considered a medical emergency; the coronary circulation is deteriorating, suddenly becoming inadequate. It must not be ignored; immediate medical attention is necessary.

Time is of the essence. If unable to reach a doctor for advice or instruction, the sufferer should immediately call for emergency help by telephone or get to the nearest hospital emergency room by the fastest means. Don't wait!

WHEN CHEST PAIN ISN'T HEART RELATED

While not all heart attacks are associated with chest pains, it is also true that not all chest pain is due to a heart attack or heart failure.

Chest pain may be due to a variety of medical problems other than coronary artery disease. Some individuals experience chest discomfort in response to anxiety and tension, much as many people subject to unusual emotional stress and strain suffer headaches. Chest pain may originate in the muscles or bones (inflammation of the rib joints, arthritis of the spine), gastrointestinal tract (esophagitis, esophageal spasm, peptic ulcer, gall bladder disease, acute pancreatitis), and lungs (lung emboli or clots, pneumonia, cancer). Or it may be due to heart or blood vessel problems other than coronary artery disease—for example, inflammation of the heart or its enveloping sack may cause chest pain.

That said, it's worth underscoring that people should not play Russian roulette with their health and attempt to guess the true cause of their chest pain. Take no chances. If you have chest pain—of any degree or variety—let a medical professional determine if it's heartburn or angina (or something else).

WHY NO CHEST PAIN

Let's end this chapter with the eight-hundred-pound gorilla in the room: Why don't the many millions of people with silent heart disease experience any chest pains?

The short answer, after thirty years of research, is that we still don't know. But we do have clues. Some people simply may not feel any pain possibly because of certain painkilling substances mysteriously produced within their bodies. Others may be suffering from long-standing damage to nerve endings that occurs more frequently in diabetics, those with chronic kidney disease, or hypertensives (sufferers of high blood pressure), three groups with a disproportionally high incidence of silent and/ or symptomatic heart attacks.

Still others actually do suffer symptoms of a heart attack—just not the gripping chest pain of angina that has been depicted repeatedly in popular culture. (Hollywood loves a good heart attack with lots of angina!) A famous country musician who was my patient had brushed aside his occasional bouts of intense heartburn—sometimes lasting a day or more—as nothing more than too much barbeque. Another patient, a much-in-demand indoor cycling instructor, could not figure out why she could lead a class up a virtual hill one week with no problem and then the next week felt completely winded on the same ride. Both of their examinations revealed silent heart disease, which they had probably suffered with for years before coming to see me.

Bottom line: If something doesn't make sense or feel right, even if you can't quite put your finger on it, have it checked by your doctor. Detection is the first step in receiving treatment for silent heart disease and the prevention of heart attacks.

4

HEART DAMAGE: STUNNING
AND CARDIAC ARREST

Now for some good news. Just a few short decades ago, surviving an acute heart attack was essentially a fifty-fifty proposition, with half of victims dying with a few days. Doctors had only the vaguest idea of the physiology underlying heart attacks, and the treatment was pretty much let the body try to heal itself and hope for the best.

Today, 90 percent of all heart attack victims survive. And except in the most extreme cases, they can go on to live long and prosper, because early detection and treatment of complications are the rule rather than the exception.

Indeed, as we learned earlier in Part I, until recently myocardial ischemia (inadequate coronary blood flow) had been considered an all-or-none process. Heart damage was known to occur if the ischemia was prolonged or severe (that is, a heart attack). But if the episode was only transient or brief (mild angina or silent myocardial ischemia), the effects on the heart were often found to be only minimal in degree and usually completely reversible. Also, it was found that after coronary flow had been restored, metabolism and function would rapidly return to normal, and heart structure would usually be preserved. Inadequate coronary artery blood flow was considered an event that simply began with a particular kind of severe chest pain (angina) and ended after the coronary blood flow had returned to normal and the chest pain had subsided.

We now know that, in most instances, angina and even a heart attack are the final—not the first—expression of heart disease. New understanding of the biochemical and physiologic effects of reduced coronary artery blood flow has led us to the conclusion that any reduction of the usual blood supply to the heart, whether intermittent or prolonged, whether painful or not, may be the beginning of a cascade of abnormal events.

In this chapter, we learn how silent heart disease can damage the heart.

THE STUNNED HEART

The first response of the oxygen-deprived heart is to malfunction in its pumping action, which is not necessarily followed by electrocardiographic changes or chest pain.

Late in the process, and virtually always only after the pumping and electrocardiographic abnormalities have developed, chest discomfort (angina) will occur in a small percentage of instances; more commonly, chest pain does not occur, and the ischemia (poor coronary blood flow) is then called silent myocardial ischemia (SMI). Thus, the ischemic cascade always begins with poor coronary artery blood flow (for the heart's needs at that moment), resulting in heart muscle malfunction, followed, on occasion, by electrocardiographic changes. Finally, in the minority of instances, this series of events is concluded with chest pain or discomfort; angina is usually the late or final expression of the ischemic cascade, not the beginning one.

The concept of the ischemic cascade helps us to understand why completely silent (or, less frequently, painful) episodes of diminished coronary artery blood flow can result in completely symptom-free, transient (or permanent), significant injuries to the heart muscle itself. These recurrent injuries may eventually diminish the pumping capacity of the heart, whether or not chest discomfort has ever occurred during any of these episodes.

Since silent episodes of heart ischemia are at least three times more frequent than painful ones, and since chest pain is usually a late feature of the ischemic cascade, significant damage to the heart's pumping abilities may occur long before chest pains develop. In other words, by the time patients start to complain of chest pains, they almost always are already afflicted with disturbed heart function of a more intense degree than appears on the surface.

Vigorous and effective treatment is therefore absolutely necessary to prevent not just the obvious episodes characterized by chest pain but, more importantly, to stop the ischemic cascade from beginning, thus giving your doctor time to take medical action to prevent temporary or permanent malfunction of the heart muscle itself and to prevent sudden death.

It was previously thought that (1) when the heart's oxygen balance was restored before permanent injury (heart attack) occurred, heart function returned rapidly to normal, and (2) when the blood flow to the heart was diminished and prolonged beyond a critical point, irreversible heart damage occurred, and, as a result, complete recovery of its pumping function could never be restored. It has now been clearly demonstrated that periods of ischemia (inadequate coronary artery blood flow), even if too brief to cause heart damage, may nevertheless be associated with profound structural and biochemical changes that will result in diminished function of the heart as a pump. This dysfunction has been found to persist for prolonged periods—hours, days, or even weeks after the blood flow has been restored.

In other words, if a heart is "stunned" by even a brief episode of ischemia, lasting hours or in some cases even just minutes, prolonged impairment of the pumping ability of the heart may result. Stunning will occur whether or not chest pain is associated with the episode of poor coronary blood flow, and therefore three to four episodes of pain-free stunning may occur for every ischemic episode associated with chest pain.

Temporary blockage of a coronary artery produces SMI or angina; complete blockage will cause a heart attack, usually with resulting permanent damage of heart muscle. But if the artery is opened quickly— with nitroglycerine, spontaneous relaxation of the coronary artery spasm, dissolution of the clot, bypass surgery, or angioplasty—before permanent damage occurs, the heart will only be temporarily stunned. It then "hibernates," waiting to recover its full function. The duration of the stunning effect is always much longer than the duration of the episode of poor blood flow; if permanent damage has not occurred, return of normal heart function will take place, but usually many hours or days after the episode of previously inadequate coronary artery blood flow has been improved.

The heart's functional ability will therefore be only temporarily affected, and total recovery will usually be permanent unless the process starts all over again. If heart stunning occurs repeatedly because of recurrent ischemia, whether painful or pain-free, the heart may never have a chance to recover completely, and permanent heart damage will result. Damage may therefore be occurring silently in persons afflicted with silent myocardial ischemia.

It may also be occurring silently and progressively in patients even with mild angina, which in the past has inappropriately been considered a minor symptom by both patients and their doctors. Eventually, repeat stunning may result in ischemic cardiomyopathy, a condition in which heart function is altered and severe heart failure may occur whether or not chest pain occurs. Patients with this condition are at greater risk of heart attack or even sudden death, so treatment must be immediate and vigorous.

Since chest pain is not a reliable guide, all episodes of ischemia, silent or not, should be treated. Only in this way can stunning be avoided. If stunning does occur, coronary artery flow should be restored as quickly as possible in order to avoid permanent damage. If the circulation is restored, the stunned heart will "hibernate" and then quite probably will be restored to normal function in time.

ISCHEMIC CASCADE

Inadequate coronary artery blood flow can have four distinct results:

1. Transient ischemia with or without chest discomfort, electrocardiographic changes, and disturbed heart function (a category that includes patients with typical angina)
2. Severe ischemia causing heart damage and permanent heart dysfunction (i.e., a classic heart attack)
3. Heart stunning consisting of abnormal function in the heart's pumping activities as a result of prolonged ischemia
4. Severe persistent heart dysfunction secondary to chronic (days, months, or years) inadequate coronary artery blood flow with resultant extremely poor (albeit usually recoverable) heart function

If heart damage has not occurred, heart function can be improved with drugs or revascularization, including surgery and angioplasty. In a significant number of instances, chest pains do not occur even when the coronary artery blood flow has been critically reduced to the point where either electrocardiographic or profound mechanical pumping abnormalities result. Angina occurs on the average in only 16 to 25 percent of these episodes and even less frequently in patients who are diabetic or hypertensive.

A malfunction of the pumping activity of the heart occurs first in response to inadequate coronary artery blood flow, followed by electrocardiographic abnormalities, which may then be followed on occasion by chest pain. Repeated stunning of the heart by ischemic episodes, silent or painful, results in permanent damage to the heart. In many instances, however, the damage may not be permanent, the heart will only be "hibernating," and function will improve if circulation can be restored.

All episodes of ischemia should be vigorously treated to prevent permanent damage. The untoward effects of repeated ischemia can be avoided or diminished in intensity if these episodes, whether painful or silent, can be reduced or eliminated.

SUDDEN CARDIAC DEATH

As we've just discussed, an episode of restricted blood flow to the heart doesn't necessarily have to result in permanent damage. Rather, the heart can merely be stunned and then hibernate until it heals itself. That's not the case with sudden cardiac arrest, which usually results in permanent heart damage and death, or sudden cardiac death.

Sudden cardiac arrest is the largest cause of natural death in the United States, causing about 325,000 adult deaths each year and responsible for half of all heart disease deaths. Only approximately 10 percent survive a sudden cardiac arrest, and only 8 percent of those will survive with good neurologic function.

Sudden cardiac arrest is not a heart attack, but the two are closely related. Heart attacks are caused by restricted blood flow to the heart, causing impaired functioning, but the heart usually keeps beating and the person remains conscious. In sudden cardiac arrest the heart stops functioning completely. Most heart attacks do not lead to cardiac arrest, but when cardiac arrest occurs, heart attack is a common cause. And, by the way, there are other causes of sudden death besides cardiac. The cessation of heart function also can be caused by trauma, drowning, drug overdose, asphyxia, and severe blood loss, to name a few. However, by far the most common cause of sudden death is heart related, caused by cardiac rhythm malfunction.

These totally unexpected cardiac-related deaths occur usually within one hour of the onset of symptoms. The usual cause of sudden death is an abnormal heart rhythm called ventricular fibrillation, which, if not promptly treated, causes death within three to four minutes. This chaotic rhythm consists of a completely disorganized quivering pattern of pumping activity resulting from attempts by many parts of the heart to contract simultaneously; the heart looks and acts like a beached jellyfish.

Coordinated contraction is impossible, and as a result pumping of blood from the heart into the circulatory system ceases. When this abnormal rhythm is found to be present in a coronary care unit, an emergency room, or even by a trained paramedic in the field, it frequently can be restored to normal rhythm using a defibrillator, a device that sends a controlled electric shock to the heart and is now required on all U.S. airlines and frequently found in other public places, including concert halls, shopping malls, and even restaurants.

Sudden death increases in frequency with increasing age, even though symptoms suggestive of heart trouble may never have been present. The peak incidence occurs between ages seventy-five and eighty-four. It is four times more common in men than in women, possibly because men do not have the same protection from coronary artery disease enjoyed by premenopausal women. Approximately half of the people who die from cardiac arrest have previously suffered heart attacks (frequently silent), and only 20 to 27 percent of the episodes are caused by a new heart attack.

A U.S. Public Health Service study conducted among the residents of the town of Framingham, Massachusetts, since 1948 reports sudden death as the first symptom or event in about 20 percent of all coronary heart disease patients. Think of what that means: one in every five people who ever develop a heart problem will die suddenly as the first expression of their heart disease; they will never know what hit them, never even suspecting that they had a heart problem. During the first thirty years of the Framingham study, half the men and almost two-thirds of the women who died suddenly had no previous history of coronary heart disease.

While sudden cardiac arrest disproportionally affects the elderly, it does strike the middle-aged. And while the frequency of these episodes in youthful athletes in the United States is extremely rare, upward of six thousand Americans aged eighteen or under die each year from sudden cardiac arrest, including young athletes (about one in fifty thousand).

Although accidents, suicide, or drugs are the most frequent overall causes of death in persons under the age of thirty, abnormalities of the heart or blood vessels are the usual cause of youthful sudden death. Persons over the age of thirty who die suddenly, whether athletic or sedentary, usually have previously been totally symptom-free and, in the vast majority of instances, are found to have arteriosclerotic heart disease, premature aging of the coronary arteries due to atherosclerosis (with resultant narrowing and/or complete blockage of these important vessels).

Patients who die suddenly, whether or not risk factors have been identified or treated, may have significant symptoms that precede the event and should alert both the patient and his or her doctor to the increased risk of sudden death. Unfortunately, many of these early symptoms are vague and nonspecific.

Earlier, we learned that Jim Fixx, the famous marathon runner and author, died quite suddenly and unexpectedly at age fifty-two. His death was quite likely caused by ventricular fibrillation, a malfunction of the heart's rhythm due to sudden inadequacy of coronary artery blood flow.

Now fast-forward to 2017, when rock star Tom Petty died suddenly and unexpectedly, just a few days after performing a sold-out concert at the Hollywood Bowl in Los Angeles. Like Fixx, who died at fifty-two, Petty's death at sixty-six was premature as well. Neither had a history of heart disease.

The difference is that while Fixx's sudden death probably was heart related (cardiac), Petty's was most likely caused by an accidental overdose of painkillers, which then caused his heart to stop functioning. Fixx's condition would be easily detected with today's diagnostics and likely reversed with today's treatment regimens. Petty's death was largely unpredictable except for the fact that there is a long history of famous entertainers experiencing sudden death from accidental overdoses, including Judy Garland and Michael Jackson.

Even though as many as 33 percent of heart attack victims consult a physician because of new or increasing chest pains in the six months before the heart injury occurs, chest pain is a relatively infrequent symptom, occurring in no more than 10 percent of sudden death cases. Shortness of breath, weakness or fatigue, chest palpitations, and a variety of other relatively imprecise complaints—such as indigestion, back pain, pain in the shoulders, arms, or hands, and so forth—occur more frequently; even though vague, these symptoms frequently are of sufficient intensity to bring the patient to a physician days or weeks prior to the final event. As many as 46 percent of sudden death victims had preexisting complaints severe enough to have caused them to see a physician within four weeks prior to death. In fact, many of these patients visited their doctor only three to four hours prior to the event!

DELAY AND DENIAL ARE DEADLY

Because significant treatable abnormalities of heart rhythm were detected prior to the occurrence of sudden death in approximately 85 percent of the out-of-hospital survivors, patients should consult their physicians as soon as possible after the onset of any significant symptoms. There really just isn't any excuse for not seeing your doctor once the red flag of symptoms is raised.

The greatest psychological danger to a patient with an acute heart attack or premonitory symptoms of sudden death is denial. Negation of personal danger by denial, one of the most common human reactions to situations of life stress, is similar to rationalization; that is, it is a patient's unconscious attempt to minimize or eliminate the threat to his or her life or health. Denial leads to an average delay (the time interval from the onset of symptoms to the arrival at a medical facility) of between 2.9 and 5.1 hours.

The enormity of this problem becomes apparent when one realizes that at least 50 percent of all deaths from heart attacks occur within four hours of the onset of symptoms, usually before the patient reaches the hospital. The size of the heart attack (and therefore the severity of subsequent complications) appears to relate to delay in treatment; patients simply do not get to well-equipped medical facilities in time to prevent or treat major problems.

Those who recognize the true cause of their symptoms will get to the hospital sooner than those who explain away their symptoms as being due to a stomachache or muscle spasm. Ironically, husbands and wives are responsible for producing more delay than are friends, associates, or employers. Denial and delay must be avoided if the incidence of sudden death is to be reduced.

Specific drug and other treatments that can reduce or often completely eliminate the potential for sudden death are available to patients who present themselves quickly enough to a hospital emergency room. Chest pain of new onset, any change (in either frequency or intensity) in a long-standing pattern of chest discomfort, or even atypical chest symptoms known as "anginal equivalents" (pains occurring in the teeth, jaw, neck, shoulders, back, arms, elbows, or fingers) should cause one to seek immediate medical attention. Also, even vague symptoms such as shortness of breath, weakness, or fatigue, as well as recurrent palpitations, should not be ignored, especially if precipitated by minimal exertion.

Physicians should be consulted as frequently as is necessary to evaluate symptoms and answer questions, especially by persons who are at high risk. Prevention and treatment of abnormal risk factors, which we'll explore in Part II of the book, will effectively reduce the incidence of sudden death.

One final note about sudden cardiac death. As with silent heart disease in general and nonfatal heart attacks, the vast majority of scientific studies have clearly demonstrated the peak onset of sudden death occurs between 6 a.m. and 12 p.m. The Massachusetts Department of Public Health and the Framingham Heart Study reported similar data. In addition, the latter group noted that the risk of sudden cardiac death was at least 70 percent greater between 7 a.m. and 9 a.m.

PART I: TAKEAWAYS

So, what did we learn in Part I? Chapter 1 discussed how the heart is a magnificent biologic pump endowed by nature with built-in redundancy. That's good news because when a silent heart disease episode strikes, unknown to its victim, in most instances the heart can partially or fully recover. However, because the human heart cannot be replaced—even with today's advanced medical technology—we must do everything we can to preserve it, to prevent damage, and, if damage does occur, to limit the size of the injury.

In Chapter 2, we discussed how most coronary heart problems are caused by narrowing or complete blockage of the coronary arteries by arteriosclerotic plaque, largely made up of excess cholesterol. Silent heart disease, an especially pernicious form of coronary heart disease because the usual warning signs often don't exist, affects up to 45 percent of heart disease sufferers. The notion that heart attacks are caused by too much physical exertion has been disproven by research. You're just as likely to suffer heart damage from silent heart disease when you're resting as when you are exercising. However, we do know that because of the body's circadian rhythm, heart events—silent and otherwise—are more likely to occur between 6 a.m. and 12 noon.

As we learned in Chapter 3, there are four types of silent heart disease. One group of patients can have cardiac strain or damage with warning signs like chest pain sometimes and at other times without any warning signs at all. In all cases, the absence of pain doesn't mean silent heart disease is benign. We don't know why about half of all those who have heart disease never experience symptoms like chest pain. The good news is that with today's modern diagnostic technology, virtually all heart disease—silent or otherwise—can be detected and treated.

43

Finally, in Chapter 4 the various kinds of heart damage caused by silent heart disease were compared. A heart "stunned" by repeated episodes of silent heart disease nevertheless can recover in some instances by, in effect, hibernating. Temporary blockage of the heart's all-important arteries need not result in permanent damage, especially if treatment is delivered quickly. The good news is that today 90 percent of all heart attack victims survive. Contrast that with sudden cardiac arrest, which kills 90 percent of its victims. It's the leading cause of death for those who suffer from heart disease and often the final result of silent heart disease damage accumulating over years. Still, sudden cardiac death can be prevented when the symptoms are recognized and treatment is provided quickly.

Now, on to Part II, where we'll explore the various risk factors associated with silent heart disease.

Part II

RISK FACTORS:
NATURE VERSUS NURTURE

PART II: INTRODUCTION

The question of which are the most important risk factors in developing silent heart disease comes down to a simple proposition: nature versus nurture, which is a shorthand way of saying genetic and inherited factors, or what you're born with, versus environmental factors, or things that have to do primarily with your lifestyle circumstances and choices.

The answer to the simple question of what is nature and what is nurture, however, is messy. If only it were as easy as labeling this risk factor as inherited and that one as caused by lifestyle habits and routines (conscious or unconscious). Take, for example, the risk factor of high low-density lipoprotein (LDL) cholesterol (the bad kind). Yes, there's a genetic component to high LDL cholesterol. If one of your parents had it, you're at an increased risk for having the condition too, and even more so if both parents had it. On the other hand, lifestyle choices play a key role in whether you actually develop it at all or to what degree it manifests in your life. The same is true for high blood pressure, diabetes, and chronic kidney disease—all high-risk factors for developing silent heart disease (and coronary artery heart disease in general).

On the other hand, take a condition like obesity. There's no doubt that lifestyle choices contribute to unhealthy excess weight, including eating a diet high in fat, sugar, and salt, not to mention living a sedentary lifestyle. Yet there appears to be an inherited component to obesity. Studies of identical twins—those rare human beings who are genetic clones of one another and make the perfect subjects for human medical studies—have shown that even twins raised in separate households with radically different diets and lifestyles tend to have excess weight if one or both biological parents were overweight.

The same is true for substance abuse. Research in the last decade has indicated that there is a genetic component to drug and alcohol addiction. Yet, undeniably, lifestyle choices contribute to the eventual outcome of whether someone at risk actually succumbs to the disease of addiction. Things get really messy when you also ask how much the genetic component of addiction is influenced when an individual is raised in a household in which one or both parents were addicts. When parents consume drugs or alcohol excessively in front of their kids and the kids later become addicts, is nature or nurture at work?

Interestingly, Swedish researchers a few years ago took a crack at the nurture-versus-nature risk factors of heart disease. In a comprehensive study, they examined the health records of all 80,214 children born in Sweden after 1931 who were adopted, along with the records of their biological parents and their adopted parents. The results? Adoptees were more likely to have had a heart attack, angina (chest pain), or another manifestation of clogged coronary arteries if they had a biological parent with one of these conditions than if an adoptive parent did. The odds were even higher if both biological parents had heart disease. Score one for nature.

But that's Sweden. The United States is a vastly bigger nation with much greater disparity in wealth, a far more ethnically diverse population, a vastly different and differentiated geography (physical environment), and a markedly less healthy diet (for the average resident). To paint the difference in broad strokes, Swedes rank twelfth among the nations of the world in overall life expectancy, with its citizens enjoying an average life expectancy of eighty-one years; the United States ranks fortieth, with an average life expectancy of seventy-seven years. As for obesity rates among its citizens, Sweden ranks twenty-first, with 9.7 percent of its total population classified as clinically obese; the United States ranks first (sigh!), with a 30.6 percent obesity rate. Even when considering access to health care as measured by the number of physicians per 1,000 people, there's a vast chasm between the two nations, with Sweden ranked fourteenth (3.3 per 1,000 persons) and the United States ranked thirty-first (2.3 per 1,000 persons). Are we comparing Swedish apples with American oranges (so to speak)?

In Part II, we boldly cross the DMZ of indecision and attribute the major risk factors for developing silent heart disease to either nature or nurture—with the understanding that there will be a good deal of overlap. Ultimately, your risk factors for developing silent heart disease are individualized and personal, depending on a host of factors specific to your profile. We'll create your own personalized silent heart disease score in Part IV of the book. In the meantime, in this next section of the book, we brave the world of potential risk factors—genetic and environmental.

5

FAMILY HISTORY

D oes silent heart disease run in your family? Have you even thought about it?

One of the most important risk factors for silent heart disease and heart disease in general is a family history of coronary disease, including heart attacks and sudden cardiac arrest. Medical conditions that run in a family are inherited by genes passed along from generation to generation.

In fact, a new study published by the *Journal of the American College of Cardiology* in June 2019 underscored just how important family history is as a risk factor in heart disease. The study involved research institutes in Europe and the United States, and its findings underscored the significance of genetic variants, or genetic differences both within and among populations, in the development of heart disease. The data revealed that attributable inheritable risk of heart disease was 32 percent—a significant jump from the previous estimate of 22 percent.

Interestingly, new research also reveals there is a distinct minority of individuals—scientists estimate about 5 percent of the general population—who have a genetic advantage when it comes to heart diseases. These lucky individuals have a genetic variation that actually lowers their risk factor by promoting smooth blood flow through the complex vascular intersections. (Disturbance of the flow leads to chronic local inflammation and formation of atherosclerotic lesions that cause heart attacks and strokes.)

Many different types of heart disease are genetic. Some conditions, including high blood pressure and coronary heart disease, can have an inherited component but likely have a number of different genetic components, or are polygenic, making them more difficult to detect through a DNA test.

Other inherited heart conditions are influenced by one gene (monogenic) or just a few genes, making them prime candidates for genetic testing, including the following:

- Arrhythmogenic right ventricular dysplasia
- Brugada syndrome
- Familial amyloidosis
- Familial dilated cardiomyopathy
- Hypertrophic cardiomyopathy
- Hypercholesterolemia
- Loeys–Dietz syndrome
- Long QT syndrome
- Marfan syndrome

Here's the good news for everybody. Since the completion in 2003 of the Human Genome Project, the international research study that mapped all the genes of the human anatomy, genetic testing for heart disease has become available to the public. We'll discuss how that works later in the chapter, but let's first take a look at how genes work.

HOW GENES WORK

Genes are the basic units of inheritance and are made up of chemicals called DNA. They provide instructions for cells to make proteins that carry out all body functions and form our physical characteristics. Each of us has more than twenty thousand genes, and each gene is present in two copies. One copy is inherited from your mother, and one copy is inherited from your father.

The genetic blueprint changes when a mutation occurs in one or more genes passed from generation to generation. The mutation could be caused by a random error during cell division or something new in the environment that prompts one or more genes to change, perhaps as a way of better adapting to some gradual ecological shift (for example, the advent of the Ice Age) or because of damage from some sudden, new external factor (like radiation from an atomic bomb).

Most genetic heart conditions are inherited in an autosomal dominant pattern. "Autosomal" means that both men and women are equally affected. "Dominant" means that although there are two copies of each gene, a mutation in just one copy is enough to cause disease. A person with an autosomal dominant condition has one normal copy of the gene and one copy with a mutation.

The chance of passing the abnormal copy of the gene to a child is one in two, or 50 percent. By the same token, each child has a 50 percent chance of inheriting the normal copy of the gene and having no risk of developing the condition. On average, half the members of a family with an autosomal dominant heart condition will develop the disease.

WHAT IS GENETIC TESTING AND WHAT CAN IT TELL ME?

Genetic testing is the process of taking a sample of a person's DNA to look for important changes in genes, or disease-causing mutations. Genetic testing can be used to do the following:

- Determine or confirm whether a person has inherited heart disease
- Identify the cause of heart disease in a family
- Predict which family members, beyond the assumed 50 percent, are most at risk of developing the inherited condition
- Provide options for family planning in order to try to avoid passing a disease-causing mutation to offspring

Genetic testing usually examines a panel of multiple genes known to cause the specific heart condition that is suspected as well as other conditions that have similar symptoms. The sequence of the patient's DNA is compared to the normal reference sequence. A single change in one gene is sufficient to cause disease. In some cases, two or more mutations may be responsible for causing disease in the family.

If possible, genetic testing should be performed in conjunction with a trained team with the experience and resources to counsel the family before and afterward. This helps individuals to make informed decisions and ensures that all concerned understand the results.

Typically, it can take a few weeks to a few months to get results, depending on the genetic test ordered. There are three potential test results for the initial person being tested: positive, negative, and inconclusive. Only positive testing results are helpful. The likelihood of getting a positive result varies by condition and the exact test performed.

To be clear, the genetic testing under discussion is not the same as popular consumer versions of genetic testing, such as those offered by 23andMe and Ancestry.com, which are largely focused on genealogy. While some of these services report on several genetic factors that impact heart health, such as those associated with coronary heart disease and atrial fibrillation, as well as a rare heart condition called hypertrophic cardiomyopathy, they do not offer medical diagnostic testing related to a personal or family history of a particular genetic disease.

MAPPING YOUR FAMILY TREE

The first step in trying to determine if heart disease runs in your family is to draw a family tree that shows who has and who doesn't have the condition of interest. This "pedigree" organizes information about the medical history of family members and identifies the pattern of inheritance and who is at risk for disease.

The most important person in your family tree is the member who currently has the most serious heart disease condition. We're looking for all the genes that might impact the family, so testing an apparently healthy family member might result in certain genes being overlooked, which could come back to haunt family members later on. The first-degree, or immediate, relatives (i.e., parents, siblings, and children) of the person already diagnosed with a heart condition should then be evaluated, a process called cascade screening.

Now, even if the genetic profile produces a clean bill of health, it's important to understand that this doesn't mean the individual doesn't have a heart condition. Indeed, it's the nature of silent heart disease to be "silent," or invisible, until it is detected by modern-day diagnostics.

Unfortunately, there is no genetic testing for silent heart disease per se, though the aforementioned medical conditions can contribute to it.

POSITIVE VERSUS NEGATIVE RESULTS

On its most basic level, genetic testing for heart disease is simple. Those who test positive for the disease-causing mutation are at risk of heart disease; those who test negative are not at risk. But let's dig a little deeper:

- A positive result means the testing facility is confident it has identified a gene mutation that can cause the family's heart disease. A positive result allows at-risk family members to do predictive genetic testing. Family members who carry the same gene mutation are at risk of developing the heart condition and should consult a cardiologist. These individuals are also at risk of passing the mutation on to their children, and these children should be examined.
- A negative result means that the laboratory did not find a mutation capable of causing disease in any of the genes they evaluated. This result is not definitive, because it is still possible that a genetic cause for a person's heart disease was simply not detected by the technology used or is present in a gene that was not tested. In this case it is not possible to offer specific, predictive genetic testing to at-risk family members to determine their risk of developing heart disease.
- Finally, the test results might reveal a change in a gene but not be conclusive as to whether the mutation can cause a heart condition or is simply a DNA variation that occurs randomly among the general population. Now, if other family members are tested and the same change appears, then that would indicate it is responsible, at least in part, for the family's heart condition.

It is important to recognize that even positive results cannot predict when the condition will develop or how severe it may be. Inheriting the mutation is not a guarantee that disease will develop, although it may cause the disease in many people.

Genetic testing is a rapidly developing field, so you should consult periodically with your cardiologist about new innovations that might affect your test results—either positively or negatively. And empower yourself by creating a Google search for "heart disease genetic testing." That way you'll know that you're getting the latest news about inherited heart conditions.

CONSEQUENCES OF GENETIC TESTING

First, let's clear the air on the legitimate concern those considering genetic testing for heart disease might have that the test results could be used against them by insurance companies or employers. Rest assured that the Genetic Information Nondiscrimination Act (GINA), signed into law in 2008, provides federal legal protection from the misuse of predictive genetic testing. However, GINA does not cover the areas of life insurance and long-term-care/disability insurance, though some states do have restrictions about how genetic information can be used in these areas. That is, these insurers may ask if you've secured genetic test results, and if you have and refuse to divulge them, they may not provide insurance. If you don't live in a state that protects against this privacy intrusion, then you might consider buying life insurance before undergoing genetic testing.

As for cost, medical genetic testing can range from a few hundred to several thousand dollars. As the tests have become more popular, their overall price has declined.

Genetic testing also raises emotional issues. Some might feel relieved to know once and for all whether they or their children have or have not inherited a gene mutation that puts them at risk of certain heart conditions. Remember our mantra: knowledge is power. Knowing your risk factor for heart disease can empower you to create a lifestyle that can combat the inherited risk factor.

Still, since genetic testing is a group effort, some family members may not want to know their genetic risk or may not want to share their lab results. It's their right, of course, and as we'll see in Part III, genetic testing is only one tool in a whole array of ways to diagnose heart disease.

6

AGE AND GENDER

In this chapter, we'll explore two of the most important biological factors in determining risk for silent heart disease: gender and age. Typically, a discussion of these two factors would begin with how middle-aged men are at the highest risk for heart attacks, and that's true: men are ten times more likely to have a heart attack than women prior to the age of forty-five. But for men and women ages sixty to seventy-nine, women actually have slightly more coronary heart disease than men: 70.2 percent of men versus 70.9 percent of women.

So rather than follow tradition, let's switch the focus on gender and age from men to women. Why? Because women share all the traditional risk factors for silent heart disease—high blood pressure, high blood sugar levels, high cholesterol levels, positive family history, smoking, and obesity—but also experience another subset of factors specific to them. (By the way, the terms "gender" and "sex" traditionally have been used interchangeably. For our discussion in this chapter and elsewhere in the book, we mean the biological differences between women and men when we refer to gender.)

First, however, let's bust another myth: heart disease is largely a men's disease. While it's true that heart attacks strike men at younger ages than they do women, the survival rates for women are worse. And for both sexes, heart disease is the number one killer. That might surprise many who think breast cancer must be the leading cause of death among women. However, more than two hundred thousand women die each year from heart attacks—five times as many as from breast cancer. Because women's symptoms are "atypical" (to use old-school parlance) compared to men's, they might be at least partially more susceptible to silent heart disease.

57

Medical science has a long tradition of essentially ignoring women. Until recently, human trial studies for new medications would only use men as test subjects. Such studies are the gold standard for testing the efficacy of a new drug and are required by the Food and Drug Administration before a drug is approved for sale to the public.

So, why would they do that? I mean, with women making up roughly half the population (50.8 percent to be exact), it would seem reasonable to assume that half the test subjects would be women. How about even 25 percent? It took effort to purposely exclude women from these studies. So, why do it? The most common reason given was that women are too "hormonal" (meaning that women's female hormones, like estrogen, are not found in the male anatomy), which would "confound" the findings.

At this point, I realize many women readers' jaws may have dropped wide open. On the other hand, they might not be surprised at all.

Today, medical researchers realize that excluding women from trial studies has a potentially serious impact on women's health. On the most basic level, women tend to be smaller than men, so the same prescriptive dosage for a man might not be appropriate for a woman.

Similarly, cardiologists have tended to view women's treatment through a male-centric lens. Under the microscope or on an MRI, a woman's heart may look just like a man's, but in fact there are significant differences that may affect the risk factors for a heart attack. For example, men and women physically react differently to stress. Her stress results in a rising pulse rate. His stress translates into increasing blood pressure.

A woman's heart is typically smaller than a man's, and the walls dividing the chambers are thinner. While a woman's heart pumps faster, each heartbeat is also about 10 percent less efficient than in men.

All very interesting, you might surmise, but what does that have to do with coronary heart disease and specifically silent heart disease? The answer is that gender impacts how heart disease symptoms manifest and how best to treat them.

These are the most important ways women's risk factors for heart disease differ from men's:

1. Women have more physical risk factors.
2. Women are older when they experience their first heart attack.

3. Heart attack symptoms can be different from those in men.
4. Some diagnostic tests aren't as effective in women.
5. Women take longer to receive medical care for their heart disease.
6. Women tend not to recover as well from a heart attack.
7. Hypertension is higher in older women.
8. Women have more lifestyle obstacles then men.

Let's dig a little deeper into each one.

MORE PHYSICAL RISK FACTORS

Women's bodies, by virtue of their reproductive system, are more complex than men's. There are diseases that only, or primarily, affect them, such as breast cancer, ovarian disease, and endometriosis. (Research shows that endometriosis, a painful disorder in which tissue that normally lines the inside of the uterus grows outside it, increases the risk of developing heart diseases by 400 percent in women under forty.) Speaking of breast cancer, new research indicates that women have a higher risk of heart disease after being treated with chemotherapy or radiation therapy. Additionally, many women may choose antiestrogen therapy if they have an estrogen-sensitive breast cancer, and loss of estrogen may be associated with higher risk of heart disease. With 3.1 million women estimated to develop invasive breast cancer each year, this poses a significant health risk for the nation. Finally, women with diabetes are at greater risk of heart disease than men with diabetes.

AGE DIFFERENCE

On average, women are five to ten years older than men when they have their first heart attack. It's thought that the female hormone estrogen is protective of women to some degree. Consequently, their risk of heart attack increases with menopause, and there's virtually no difference between men and women's risk of heart attack by age seventy. At first glance, that might seem a distinct advantage for women, but it comes with its own risk. Heart attacks in younger, premenopausal women can be missed by the women themselves and their physicians because they are relatively uncommon. In fact, every year in the United States, heart disease kills sixteen thousand women ages thirty to fifty-five and results in forty thousand hospitalizations.

DIFFERENT SYMPTOMS

Studies suggest that women are more likely to have a wider range of symptoms not typically associated with heart attacks. The classic symptoms of chest pain and crushing pressure or weight are simply absent in many women with an acute heart attack. Instead, women have different symptoms that are often shared with other afflictions, such as sudden and dramatic fatigue, excessive sweating, and pain in the neck, back, or jaw—symptoms that might be misdiagnosed as associated with lupus, menopause, or stress.

DIFFICULTY IN DIAGNOSIS

Heart disease can be more difficult to diagnose in women. An angiogram is among the most effective and widely used X-ray tests for finding blockages in the heart's arteries and a key diagnostic tool in determining and preventing silent heart disease. But coronary heart disease in women, more often than in men, affects small arteries, which are more difficult to see in X-rays.

DELAYED MEDICAL CARE

In a recent study of fifty people age sixty-five and older, researchers found that women hospitalized for heart disease were less likely to receive beneficial medications, including everything from the most basic, like aspirin, to the latest cholesterol-lowering pharmaceuticals. Research also shows women tend to arrive in emergency rooms later than men, after heart damage already has occurred. Again, their so-called atypical symptoms may be at play here, with women downplaying or misinterpreting warning signs of an acute heart event.

LESS SUCCESSFUL RECOVERY

Women who suffer a heart attack on average require longer hospitalization than men and are more likely to die before leaving the hospital. Social-psychological factors may be at work here: perhaps it's a reflection of women putting their families' health and welfare before their own. Or the reasons may have more to do with other untreated illnesses more prevalent in women than men, including diabetes and high blood pressure. Or it may be the case that women don't receive the right medications. We know, for example, that women have a greater risk of developing a blood clot following heart attacks yet are less likely to be given drugs to prevent blood clots.

HYPERTENSION

More than 45 percent of U.S. adults have high blood pressure or hypertension, a leading risk factor for silent heart disease. While hypertension is lower among young women compared to men of the same age, the reverse is true for the elderly.

LIFESTYLE CHALLENGES

We often think of depression as affecting mainly the brain. But new research is showing that depression can increase inflammation, in turn leading to *atherosclerosis* or blockage of the arteries. Women's hearts seem to be more impacted than men's by depression. Stress and depression can also make it more difficult to maintain a healthy lifestyle regimen, such as following treatments, eating a healthy diet, or getting a good night's sleep. Smoking is detrimental to everyone's health, but in women smoking poses a greater risk factor for heart disease than in men. Some studies even indicate that a sedentary lifestyle is more of a risk factor for heart disease in women than in men.

AGE AS A RISK FACTOR

Now let's turn to another major risk factor for silent heart disease: aging. People age sixty-five and older are much more likely than younger people to suffer a heart attack, to have a stroke, or to develop coronary heart disease (commonly called heart disease) and heart failure.

Aging can cause changes in the heart and blood vessels. As you get older, your heart doesn't beat as fast during physical activity or during fight-or-flight times of stress. However, your heart rate (the number of heartbeats per minute) at rest does not change significantly with normal aging.

As we learned earlier, a major cause of heart disease is the buildup of fatty deposits in the walls of arteries over many years. The good news is there are things you can do to delay, lower, or possibly negate or reverse your risk.

The most common aging change is increased stiffness, or hardening, of the arteries. In turn, this causes high blood pressure, or hypertension, which can further damage the heart, and so a downward spiral of cause and effect begins.

Age can cause other changes to the heart:

- Age-related changes in the electrical system can lead to arrhythmias—a rapid, slowed, or irregular heartbeat—and/or the need for a pacemaker.
- Valves—the one-way, door-like parts that open and close to control blood flow between the chambers of your heart—may become thicker and stiffer. Stiffer valves can limit the flow of blood out of the heart and become leaky.
- The chambers of an aging heart often increase in size. As the heart wall thickens, the amount of blood that a chamber can hold diminishes, despite the increased overall heart size. The heart may fill more slowly.

- Long-standing hypertension can cause an increased thickness of the heart wall, which can increase the risk of atrial fibrillation, a common heart rhythm problem in older people.
- As we get older, we become more sensitive to salt, which may cause an increase in blood pressure and/or ankle or foot swelling (edema).

TAKEAWAY

So, age and gender are both significant factors in the risk of developing silent heart disease.

One more thing: I would be remiss if I didn't conclude this chapter with a final comment about aging. Generally, the older you are, the higher risk you have of coronary heart disease, and the majority of people who die of coronary heart disease are sixty-five or older. That's been dogma ever since the medical profession began observing heart disease centuries ago.

But in a new study released in May 2019 by the Centers for Disease Control and Prevention (CDC) and the U.S. Department of Health and Human Services, more middle-aged people today are dying from heart disease than in recent years, reversing a decade-long trend that witnessed heart disease rates declining for all age groups.

Experts believe the reason for this disturbing development is that rates of obesity, diabetes, and a sedentary lifestyle—all risk factors for heart disease—are going up for this age group. (We will explore all these factors in coming chapters.) But also, adults ages forty-five to sixty-four today are less likely to have medical insurance than they were ten years ago as more working- and middle-class Americans simply can't afford it. Seniors tend to be immune to the health impact of stagnant wages and the lingering effects of the Great Recession, since they have guaranteed health care through Medicare.

7

HIGH LDL CHOLESTEROL

In the long history of understanding, diagnosing, and treating heart disease, the Framingham study of 1948 remains a benchmark. Before the study, despite decades of research and observation, doctors didn't know what caused heart disease or why people were dying from heart attacks.

What was known was that "diseases of the heart" had become the leading cause of death among Americans, killing more than 460,000 in 1948 alone. To frame it another way, 418,000 Americans (mostly soldiers) died during World War II in or as a result of combat. In the three years after the war, heart disease had killed more than three times as many Americans—and the rate of death was increasing at an alarming clip.

A group of medical researchers proposed a definitive longitudinal (over time) study of people to determine once and for all the factors behind the epidemic of heart disease. The researchers chose the town of Framingham, Massachusetts, because it was close to their research centers based in Boston. The town was chosen not because it was special but instead because its population profile seemed to match that of most of the country: it had a foundation of longtime residents, a fairly recent infusion of new immigrants, and an emerging middle class.

In 1948, Framingham had a population of about 28,000. Remarkably, 5,209 residents volunteered for the original heart study, which, by the way, continues today with 15,000 volunteers from a population of 63,000, including many who are first- and second-generation offspring of the original volunteers.

When the study began, what seem today to be such obvious risk factors for coronary artery heart disease—for example, the correlation between cigarette smoking and high blood pressure—were still unknown. Incredibly, some medical professionals believed an elevated blood pressure might even be good for you. The eminent U.S. cardiologist Paul Dudley White in 1937 suggested that "hypertension may be an important compensatory mechanism which should not be tampered with, even if we were certain that we could control it." By the 1950s many doctors still thought that unless it was severe, hypertension was a relatively benign condition.

Equally incredible was the popular notion that filtered, versus non-filtered, cigarettes lowered the risk of heart disease. (That wasn't definitively disproven by the Framingham study until the 1970s.)

But of all the results of the famed Framingham study, none were more important than its findings about cholesterol and specifically that high levels of low-density lipoprotein (LDL) cholesterol may be a major cause of clogged and narrowed arteries (arteriosclerosis). Before Framingham, it was generally thought these conditions were normal parts of aging, occurring universally as people became older, and there was nothing much to be concerned about. After Framingham, researchers could clearly see from the data that the volunteers who had high LDL cholesterol levels also had the highest incidence of heart disease and suffered the most from its severest forms, including heart attack and cardiac arrest. It's because of the Framingham volunteers and the research team who studied them that we now know that people with high cholesterol have about twice the risk of heart disease as people with lower (normal) levels of cholesterol and LDL.

CAUSES OF HIGH LDL CHOLESTEROL

Cholesterol is a waxy, fat-like substance. Your body needs some cholesterol. It's essential for making the cell membrane and cell structures and is vital for synthesis of hormones, vitamin D, and other substances, but it can build up on the walls of your arteries and lead to arterial heart disease and stroke when you have too much in your blood.

Low-density lipoprotein cholesterol is known as bad cholesterol (because it clogs the arteries). High-density lipoprotein (HDL) cholesterol is known as good cholesterol (because it's essential for cell membrane synthesis), and high HDL levels in the blood are associated with fewer heart attacks and strokes.

High blood cholesterol is a condition that causes the levels of certain bad fats, or lipids, to be too high in the blood. This condition is usually caused by lifestyle factors, notably diet, but as we learned in the last chapter, heart disease can be inherited, and so can a proclivity for higher than normal LDL cholesterol levels. Genetic studies have found that related family members tend to have similar levels of LDL and HDL cholesterol. Less commonly, high cholesterol is caused by other medical conditions or some medicines.

The Framingham findings were so important because the problem of excessive cholesterol, which leads to clogged arteries, is pervasive: nearly one in every three Americans has LDL cholesterol levels that are unhealthy. That is, more than 102 million American adults (age twenty or older) have total cholesterol levels at or above 200 mg/dL, which is above healthy levels. More than 35 million of these people have levels of 240 mg/dL or higher, which puts them at higher risk for heart disease. Combine this with high levels of triglycerides, the most common type of body fat, and, well, then you have the recipe for heart attack, stroke, and silent heart disease.

Use the chart in table 7.1 to determine with your doctor whether your cholesterol levels are safe.

Table 7.1.

Desirable Cholesterol Levels	
Total cholesterol	Less than 200 mg/dL
LDL ("bad" cholesterol)	Less than 100 mg/dL
HDL ("good" cholesterol)	60 mg/dL or higher
Triglycerides	Less than 150 mg/dL

Here's the kicker to the whole problem of cholesterol: Like silent heart disease itself, high blood cholesterol does not cause specific symptoms. However, your doctor can do a simple blood test to check your levels. The National Cholesterol Education Program recommends that adults get their cholesterol checked every five years.

CHOLESTEROL FROM FOOD

Within the cells, cholesterol is the precursor molecule in several bio-chemical pathways. For example, in the liver, cholesterol is converted into bile, which is then stored in the gallbladder. Bile is made up of bile salts, which help in making the fats more soluble and easier to absorb. Several animal fats are sources of cholesterol. Animal fats are complex mixtures of triglycerides and contain lower amounts of cholesterols and phospholipids.

Major dietary sources of cholesterol include cheese, egg yolks, beef, pork, poultry, and shrimp. Cholesterol is not found in plant-based foods; however, plant products such as flax seeds and peanuts may contain cholesterol-like compounds called phytosterols, which are beneficial and actually help in lowering cholesterol levels.

Saturated fats and trans fats in food are the worst culprits in raising blood cholesterol. Saturated fats are present in full-fat dairy products, animal fats, several types of oil, and chocolate. Trans fats are present in hydrogenated oils. These do not occur in significant amounts in nature and are found mainly in fast foods, snack foods, and fried or baked goods.

We'll take an even deeper dive into the differences between satu-rated and unsaturated fats in Chapter 10.

NEXT-GENERATION CHOLESTEROL

Now, before we close, we'll tackle one more myth about high-choles-terol levels: it's only a problem for adults. While it's true that the vast majority of those who suffer from high LDL cholesterol are adults with a skew toward middle-aged and older adults, increasingly we're finding the problem is affecting youth.

Two recent studies published in the *Journal of the American Medical Association* found that heart disease risk factors—including elevated LDL cholesterol levels—increasingly were showing up in children. Additional research compiled in the Bogalusa Heart Study found that childhood cholesterol measurements predicted future artery thickness.

The Bogalusa Heart Study is like the Framingham Heart Study in that both have tested a population over several decades, but it is different in several important ways. First, the town of Bogalusa in southern Louisiana is racially mixed between whites and blacks, while Framingham was almost entirely white. Second, the study purposefully includes children. Finally, the population studied is largely rural (versus Framingham's suburban population), and it is the only controlled, longitudinal study of its kind located in the South.

Headed by Tulane University medical professor Gerald Berenson, MD, the team of researchers began collecting data in 1972, making it the longest-running biracial health study in the world. The study has generated thousands of peer-reviewed articles. "We started our study with school-age children, from 5 to 17 years old. Because of the results we went down to preschool age, 2.5 to 5.5 years old," said Berenson in an interview in *Global Health Magazine*. Ultimately, the Bogalusa team sought birth records to try to answer questions about birth weight and risk of heart disease and diabetes. A majority of the people who began participating in the study as schoolchildren continued to come back to the Bogalusa clinic for follow-up health checks as first years and then decades rolled by, creating a generation of heart health data.

Key findings of the study include the following:

- The major etiologies of adult heart disease, atherosclerosis, coronary heart disease, and essential hypertension begin in childhood. Documented anatomic changes occur by five to eight years of age.
- Cardiovascular risk factors can be identified in early life.
- The levels of risk factors in childhood are different from those in the adult years. Levels change with growth phases, notably in the first year of life, during puberty and adolescence, in the transition to young adulthood, and in adulthood.
- Autopsy studies clearly indicate atherosclerosis and hypertension begin in early life.

The take-home message from Bogalusa? Adult heart disease is now beginning in childhood for many individuals, and elevated LDL cholesterol levels are a primary culprit in this new phenomenon. Dietary control of cholesterol, LDL and HDL, should be addressed at all ages.

8

HIGH BLOOD PRESSURE

To know my patient Frank is to love him. He has a big, boisterous, salesman's personality—perfect for LA's highly competitive garment industry. At forty-five years old, he's already considered an "elder" in this youth-centric business. A classic Type A, he's outgoing, ambitious, rigidly organized, highly status conscious, sensitive, impatient, anxious, proactive, and concerned with time management.

In short, Frank is a high-achieving "workaholic." He's also had several coronary events in which he felt chest pains—the classic symptom of a heart attack. But we know through the miracle of modern-day diagnostics that he has had silent heart disease for several years; diagnostic images reveal multiple scars on his heart, the telltale sign of the disease. He also has several risk factors, including a family history of heart disease and the stress and related anxiety that comes with his personality type.

But his biggest problem is hypertension, or high blood pressure. Perhaps of all the major risk factors, hypertension is the most common, affecting nearly one in two adults. What's more, it's often the "silent killer" in coronary disease, because about one in three people with high blood pressure don't even know they have it. Like silent heart disease itself, this silent killer is usually asymptomatic.

There's a standard profile for patients most at risk for hypertension: men are at greater risk than women, African Americans and South Asians have higher incidences than other groups, and the mean age for acute hypertension is sixty years old. (However, increasingly, younger adults are suffering from it; more on this later in the chapter.)

Is hypertension an inherited condition? There's likely a genetic factor to hypertension, but medical science isn't quite sure why. From numerous studies, we do know that if your parents or close blood relatives have had high blood pressure, you are at a higher risk of developing it too.

WHAT IS HYPERTENSION?

Hypertension, often referred to as high blood pressure, occurs when the force of blood against the artery walls is too high. Blood pressure, or how hard your blood is pushing against your arteries as it moves through your body, is measured using two numbers. The first number, called systolic blood pressure, measures the pressure in your blood vessels when your heart beats. The second number, called diastolic blood pressure, measures the pressure in your blood vessels when your heart rests between beats. If the measurement reads 120 systolic and 80 diastolic, you would say, "120 over 80," or write, "120/80 mmHg."

That particular measurement, 120/80 mmHg, is significant because traditionally that's been the benchmark of whether a patient has normal or healthy blood pressure. Patients with higher measurements were considered, depending on how much higher, as having prehypertension (between 120/80 and 139/89 mmHg) or bona fide hypertension (anything above 139/89 mmHg).

However, recently, the American College of Cardiology and American Heart Association task force updated guidelines for doctors and their patients with the hope of better outcomes for people at risk for or living with this condition. Released on November 13, 2017, they are the first full set of guidelines for blood pressure in the United States since 2003. The aim is to help patients reduce their risk of developing high blood pressure and improve health outcomes for those already living with it. Below are key points that every patient should know about the update.

The most important aspect of the new guidelines is that now there are four traditional blood pressure categories:

- Stage 1, or elevated blood pressure (prehypertension), is 120/80 to 139/89 mmHg.
- Stage 2, or mild hypertension, is 140/90 to 159/99 mmHg.
- Stage 3, or moderate hypertension, is 160/100 to 179/109 mmHg.
- Stage 4, or severe hypertension, is 180/110 mmHg or higher.

It's important to note that the new guidelines replace the term "prehypertension" with "elevated blood pressure." This label includes patients with an elevated blood pressure who are at higher risk for developing full-blown high blood pressure.

What's behind these changes? Research shows that adults with blood pressure readings considered prehypertensive under the old guidelines are already at up to double the risk of having a major cardiovascular event—a heart attack or stroke—compared to those with normal blood pressure. In addition, recent clinical trials have shown that lowering systolic blood pressure to 120 mmHg results in significant cardiovascular benefit in high-risk patients compared with patients with blood pressures less well controlled.

Of those who fall into the new elevated blood pressure and stage 1 categories, only a small number will need blood pressure–lowering medication. However, everyone in this group should be aggressively treating all their abnormal cardiac risk factors.

Having elevated or stage 1 high blood pressure is a red flag signaling that you must make purposeful lifestyle changes. Based on a number of studies the following changes—though not always easy—are proven to lower blood pressure, protect heart health, and also carry other health benefits: maintaining a healthy weight, eating a heart-healthy diet (which may include lowering your salt intake and boosting your potassium intake), limiting alcohol intake, and engaging in regular physical activity. We'll tackle each of these risk factors in the next section of the book.

Based on the new guidelines, gauging someone's risk for heart or vascular disease can help determine how to best manage blood pressure—that is, whether risk factor management alone will suffice or whether these therapeutic changes should be coupled with medical interventions such as cholesterol-lowering or blood pressure–controlling medications. These risk factors include age, gender, total and LDL levels, cigarette smoking, diabetes, and obesity.

Using this risk estimate helps us pinpoint who is likely to benefit most from blood pressure–lowering medications. If your risk of having a heart attack or stroke is 10 percent or higher—meaning that you have a one in ten chance of developing cardiovascular disease or more—you should be taking a blood pressure–lowering medication in addition to adopting heart-healthy lifestyle changes. Regular medical evaluation is recommended at least every one to three weeks, or until blood pressure has become well controlled.

OTHER RISK FACTORS FOR HYPERTENSION

Back to our friend, Frank. As I told him, the good news was that while hypertension is among the most serious of risk factors for silent heart disease, it's also among the most treatable. After a complete physical, he enthusiastically embraced (as only a Type A personality can!) a healthy lifestyle regimen, complete with a Mediterranean-style diet, regular exercise, and meditation to reduce his stress levels and ensure a restful night's sleep. OK, he embraced almost everything. I can still hear him now. "Aw, Doc, do I have to? Meditation is like torture to me. How about a cut back on the afternoon espressos instead?" And, oh, yes. Frank is no longer indulging in his after-lunch coffee drinks.

As I mentioned earlier, Frank is in many ways typical of those at risk for high blood pressure—male, prone to stress, with a sedentary lifestyle and unhealthful diet—but just a generation ago, he would have been considered an outlier. His demographic profile would not have been average because he would have been too young. Just ten years ago it would have been relatively uncommon for me to see a patient in his or her forties experiencing significant hypertension, but that's changing, and researchers aren't quite sure why. There seems to be a correlation between obesity and hypertension in people younger than fifty years old.

And here's the real problem: young people tend to think they're invincible, especially when it comes to a condition like high blood pressure, which they associate with parents or grandparents. But dismissing the possibility of hypertension can be a dangerous gamble. Young adults with even slightly above normal blood pressure may be more likely to have heart problems later in life, according to a new study in the *Journal of the American College of Cardiology*. The study focused on nearly twenty-five hundred men and women who were eighteen to thirty years old when the study began. Researchers kept track of them for twenty-five years, taking closer looks at the participants' health seven times. The checkups included blood pressure readings.

Near the end of the study, participants also had heart-imaging tests. Some people had slightly above normal blood pressure (120/80 to 139/89 mmHg) when they were still under age thirty. (Again, this level, which is not high enough to be considered high blood pressure, is known as elevated blood pressure or prehypertension.) But the researchers found that people with above normal blood pressure were more likely to have signs of heart disease in middle age. In particular, they were more likely to have problems with the left ventricle of the heart.

Which brings us to women. Again, the poster child for patients with dangerously high blood pressure is the aging, overweight, white male. Indeed, according to the latest research, by their mid-fifties, about one in four men and only two in five women still have normal blood pressure, and about half of men and women have a blood pressure that is above normal but not yet high enough to be considered hypertension. Studies also show that men are more prone to hypertension than women below the age of fifty. But here's the point: after the age of fifty, women are at a slightly higher risk for the disease because of menopause. To frame it another way, at sixty-five and older, women are more likely to develop high blood pressure than men.

What about younger women? Half of women who develop high blood pressure by their early forties will develop heart disease or increased risk of stroke later in life (and statistically, many of those will develop silent heart disease). Even younger women aren't immune to the dangers of high blood pressure since 7 percent of women between twenty and thirty-four have high blood pressure. While the rate is low compared to men, young women are far less likely to be diagnosed with and treated for the condition.

Bottom line: For young women and men, keeping blood pressure in check reduces the risk of stroke by 48 percent.

Let's go back to Frank one more time. His white, male archetype for high blood pressure masks another reality: high blood pressure affects people of color more than white people. In particular two groups at heightened risk for hypertension are African American adults and adults of Southeast Asian descent.

Black adults are up to two times more likely to develop high blood pressure by age fifty-five compared to whites, with many of these racial differences developing before age thirty, concluded a study recently published in the *Journal of the American Heart Association*. Known as the Coronary Artery Risk Development in Young Adults (CARDIA) Study, it tracked the blood pressure of U.S. adults from young adulthood through middle age. It included 3,890 adults between the ages of eighteen and thirty, all of whom were free of high blood pressure at baseline and followed for up to thirty years. Participants were from four U.S. cities (Birmingham, Alabama; Chicago, Illinois; Minneapolis, Minnesota; and Oakland, California) and enrolled in the study during the mid-1980s. The goal of the recent analysis was to see how many black people developed high blood pressure and at what age compared to white people, and it revealed that black participants face significantly higher rates of hypertension compared to white adults. By the end of the CARDIA Study, 75 percent of black adults had developed high blood pressure, compared to just 55 percent of white men and 40 percent of white women. Depending on a participant's initial blood pressure, this difference translated to 1.5 to 2 times greater risk for hypertension among black adults compared to white adults. Researchers noted that many of these differences developed by age thirty, highlighting the need for early intervention. The take-home message, according to the authors, is the importance of high blood pressure prevention in black people beginning at a young age.

Another study found that African Americans are also more prone to hypertensive crisis, a complication of high blood pressure in which blood pressure quickly soars to life-threatening levels. This condition is particularly dangerous because it can lead to permanent organ damage as well as heart attacks and cardiac arrest. All patients with hypertension should follow a prescriptive regimen for a healthy lifestyle and diet, but patients who have experienced a hypertensive crisis must also assiduously follow a regimen of medications as prescribed by their doctor.

While there is a foundational awareness in the black community and among medical professionals of the risk of hypertension for black adults, that's not the case with American adults of Southeast Asian descent. Generally, the medical community views Asian Americans through a single lens: that is, Asian Americans compare favorably with other ethnic groups in terms of overall health and especially when it comes to heart disease. That poses an inherent danger that both patients and their doctors will overlook high blood pressure based on implicit bias.

A published study evaluated South Asians living in the United States—3.4 million people mostly from Bangladesh, Bhutan, India, the Maldives, Nepal, Pakistan, and Sri Lanka, who make up one of the fastest-growing ethnic groups in the United States. The results reveal that this group experiences heart disease at a younger age and has higher rates of heart disease than their white counterparts. While heart disease is the leading killer of all Americans, data suggests that Southeast Asians face especially high rates of heart disease in the United States. Southeast Asians living in the United States also are at increased risk for a cluster of risk factors associated with heart disease, including hypertension as well as diabetes and high cholesterol.

Now, all the warnings about the dangers of high blood pressure discussed in this chapter might seem dire, and without a doubt, high blood pressure is a leading factor in the genesis of heart disease. Worse, the disease is widespread (with one in two adult Americans suffering from it) and "silent," without any easily recognizable symptoms. But the good news is that it's highly treatable. We have decades now of research and clinical practice that show us how changes to diet and lifestyle, together with medications when needed, can control high blood pressure.

9

DIABETES AND KIDNEY DISEASE

Angelica was a rocket scientist—literally. She worked at the famed NASA Jet Propulsion Laboratory (JPL) in Los Angeles. In a place filled with brainiacs, Angelica, an African American woman in her fifties, was among the brightest stars in the sky. She was part of the team that put the first landing rover, the *Sojourner Truth*, on Mars.

So, it was surprising that she was only now visiting me—her first-ever appointment with a cardiologist. I say that because she was fully aware that she had type 2 diabetes. What had escaped her—apparently her primary care doctor as well—was the relationship between diabetes and heart disease.

"I go to my doctor at least every six months to check my blood sugar levels," she said. "Believe me, I'm not the kind of person who takes chances. I can't in my profession. Everything at JPL is checked and rechecked. And I can assure you that I certainly don't take any chances with my health," she said.

"And your doctor never thought to check for signs of atherosclerosis?" I questioned.

"Well, no. But why should she have checked? I've never experienced chest pains or any other symptoms of heart disease," she protested.

Exactly. That is the problem. Many doctors and their patients who suffer from diabetes are not aware that cardiovascular disease is a common comorbidity of diabetes, and this correlation over the past three decades has only grown stronger.

But let's be clear: cardiologists are as big a part of the problem. Just as primary care doctors may not check for signs of atherosclerosis, many cardiologists may not check a patient's blood sugar level.

The clear association between heart disease and diabetes is a phenomenon well known by medical researchers but not so much among medical practitioners in general and even less by their patients. A survey released by the American Heart Association found that only a third of diabetics realized that heart disease was among the "most serious" complications for which they were at risk, even though almost twice that number would experience a cardiovascular problem.

So, let's state the facts once and for all: the 30.3 million adult Americans with diabetes have a risk of dying of a heart attack or stroke two to four times as great as that of someone who has already survived a heart attack. To frame it another way, at least 68 percent of people age sixty-five or older with diabetes die from some form of heart disease, and 16 percent die of stroke.

In addition to the 30.3 million Americans diagnosed with diabetes, more than twice as many—another 70 million with prediabetes (a condition characterized by slightly elevated blood glucose levels)—are also at high risk for coronary heart disease. Patients with or at high risk for diabetes and their doctors too often tend to treat heart disease as a separate concern. Worse, because silent heart disease is an asymptomatic coronary heart condition, diabetes patients and their doctors might not even consider it life threatening, despite the evidence to the contrary. While it's understandable that for persons with diabetes the focus of their medical care is the treatment of diabetes, they should never ignore their heightened risk for heart disease.

In this chapter, we'll also discuss kidney disease, which affects 37 million people in the United States (or 15 percent of adult Americans) and is the ninth leading cause of death. Like those with diabetes, people with kidney disease are also at risk for silent heart attacks—the ones that may go unnoticed—because both diseases can cause neuropathy, or damage to the peripheral nervous system. As a result, researchers believe that diabetics and kidney disease sufferers simply can't feel when they have a heart attack.

WHAT IS DIABETES?

People with diabetes cannot fully regulate their blood sugar levels, and if the disease isn't monitored constantly, blood sugar can spike to abnormally high levels, a condition called hyperglycemia, or less often dip below normal, a condition called hypoglycemia. Both conditions are potentially life threatening and can lead to coma and death if not recognized and promptly treated.

In a sense, diabetes is not one but two disorders. Type 1 diabetes, formerly known as juvenile diabetes, is an immunological disease in which a person is born without the ability to produce insulin, a hormone made in your pancreas that is essential for your body to use glucose for cellular energy. In type 2 diabetes, formerly known as adult-onset diabetes, the pancreas still makes insulin but not enough, or the insulin doesn't work in the body like it should, and blood sugar levels get too high. Another difference is that type 2 diabetes is a progressive disease and worsens over time. Eventually, most patients with prediabetes or type 2 diabetes will need to use a blood-sugar-controlling oral medication or injectable insulin (just like virtually all type 1 diabetes patients).

Both kinds of diabetes have a genetic connection. If your parents had type 1 or type 2 diabetes, you're at greater risk of developing the disease. But as is the case with heart disease, the fact that you're at a higher risk of the disease doesn't mean you will get it. Lifestyle, diet, and other environmental factors are important determinants.

Type 2 diabetes patients also commonly have a condition called insulin resistance. While they're able to make insulin, their bodies can't use it properly to move glucose into the cells. So, the amount of glucose in the blood rises. The pancreas then makes more insulin to try to overcome this problem.

But in order to develop insulin resistance and type 2 diabetes, you must also have a genetic abnormality. Along the same lines, some people with type 2 don't produce enough insulin; that is also due to a genetic abnormality. That is, not everyone can develop type 2 diabetes. Additionally, not everyone with a genetic abnormality will develop type 2 diabetes; other genetic risk factors and lifestyle choices influence the development.

Insulin resistance has a strong correlation with obesity, but scientists aren't exactly clear how it works. Indeed, when bariatric surgery became popular in the first decade of the twenty-first century as a means of treating extreme obesity, a surprising side effect in many patients with diabetes was that the disease instantly disappeared. They no longer had to take insulin. Since bariatric surgery involves several different techniques in which the capacity of the stomach is shrunk, on the face of it that should have no impact on diabetes, since insulin is produced in the pancreas. While there is no known cure for diabetes per se, bariatric surgery for some patients does, indeed, appear to cure the disease for reasons still unknown.

BEFORE AND AFTER 1921

Diabetes was well known although not well understood by the ancients, and only recently has its connection to heart disease been identified. In the history of diabetes treatment, one date stands out: everything can be categorized as falling before 1921 or afterward.

More than three thousand years ago, the Egyptians were writing about a physical condition characterized by excessive urination, thirst, and weight loss—all traits of type 1 diabetes. Around the same time Ayurvedic physicians in India identified the disease and called it *ama-dhumeha*, or honey urine, as they noted that the urine of its sufferers attracted ants. The term "diabetes," from the ancient Greek word for "to pass through," was first used in 250 BC by Apollonius of Memphis, a reference to excessive urination associated with the disease. In the fifth century AD, Chinese physicians had already figured out the two types of diabetes.

In the Middle Ages, physicians thought the disease was a condition of the kidneys, because of its association with excessive urination. Physicians treated it with a wildly imaginative array of regimens, from a diet of rancid animal foods to smoking tobacco to exercise on horseback to wearing warm flannel clothes. But give credit to the medieval doctors for discovering that metformin (known then as goat's rue or French lilac) was effective in treating diabetes. Fast-forward a few centuries, and metformin again would become available in 1995 in the United States as a treatment approved by the Food and Drug Administration for pre–type 2 diabetes.

By the late eighteenth century, English and Italian physicians, through autopsies, had observed that damage to the pancreas, not kidneys, was likely the cause of diabetes. And then came the first breakthrough in 1910, when Sir Edward Albert Sharpey-Schafer found that people with diabetes were deficient in a single chemical normally produced by the pancreas. He proposed calling this substance insulin and described the endocrine role it played in metabolism.

Then, in 1921, Frederick Grant Banting and Charles Herbert Best demonstrated that they could reverse induced diabetes in dogs by giving them an extract from the pancreases of healthy dogs. Eureka! They went on to purify the hormone insulin from bovine pancreases, and the first patient treated successfully was a fourteen-year-old boy with type 1 diabetes, Leonard Thompson, who weighed only sixty-five pounds at the time because of his disease. By 1924, insulin was in mass production and being distributed around the world. The insulin that Banting and Best developed nearly a century ago is essentially the same as is used today.

THE CARDIOVASCULAR CONNECTION

What is the link between diabetes and coronary heart disease, including asymptomatic silent heart disease? Over time, high blood glucose from type 2 diabetes can damage blood vessels and the nerves that control the heart and blood vessels. The longer one has type 2 diabetes, the greater the chances of developing heart disease.

People with type 1 diabetes are also at increased risk for heart disease, though the reasons for this are less clear. A recent study reported in the *New England Journal of Medicine* found solid evidence that aggressively lowering a person's blood sugar level can cut the risk of heart attack and stroke nearly in half, at least for type 1 diabetes. Whether stringent glucose control also halves cardiovascular disease in type 2 diabetes is being studied by the National Institutes of Health.

Type 2 diabetes and cardiovascular disease share deep molecular roots in the regulation of sugar and fat throughout the body. That relationship seems logical, because diabetes involves the way food is metabolized, a process that involves cholesterols, which can cause blood vessels to clog.

There is one positive side to the diabetes–heart disease connection. The same avoidance of risk factors for heart disease also appears to prevent or delay the onset of type 2 diabetes. A large National Institutes of Health–sponsored study, the Diabetes Prevention Program, and other studies have proven that modest weight-reduction and a thirty-minute exercise routine five days a week can reduce the development of type 2 diabetes over three years by more than 50 percent. Even people with diabetes frequently have abnormalities in blood pressure and lipid levels that can be detected and treated to prevent cardiovascular disease.

By the way, that was good news for my patient Angelica. She already was pursuing a lifestyle of moderate exercise, stress reduction (yoga, in her case), and a whole-foods diet—all good for treating diabetes and heart disease.

In the last ten years, large-scale research studies around the world have shown that optimal control of low-density lipoprotein (LDL) (the "bad" cholesterol) levels and blood pressure can prevent adverse cardiovascular outcomes by 30 to 50 percent. The American Diabetes Association and the American Heart Association recommend an LDL cholesterol goal in all adults with diabetes of less than 100 mg/dL. In people who already have heart disease, a more desirable LDL cholesterol goal should be less than 70 mg/dL, based on evidence from more recent studies. The blood pressure goal in all patients with diabetes is less than 130/80 mmHg. In most patients with diabetes, reaching these targets for blood pressure could require two or more medications. Fortunately, we have safe and effective medications available to help patients meet their lipid and blood pressure goals.

A LOOK AHEAD

Being the space scientist that she was, Angelica was interested in future treatments for patients with both diabetes and heart disease. Immunotherapy, stem cell therapy, genetic engineering, and artificial pancreases were all lines of research being pursued, I told her.

One of the most exciting developments on the near horizon is from a bioengineering team at the University of California, Los Angeles, school of medicine that has developed a type of "smart" skin patch that monitors a patient's blood sugar automatically—probably reducing the need for injections. It helps to keep blood sugar at normal levels and reduces the risk of hypoglycemia. The device has been successfully tested in the lab, and preclinical trials on humans could begin in 2020.

"You know, Dr. Karpman, you can count me in for anything that's smart," chuckled Angelica. In the meantime, we agreed to keep her diabetes *and* cardiovascular disease in check by keeping her cholesterol levels and blood pressure under control and continuing her healthy lifestyle regimen.

KIDNEY DISEASE AND SILENT HEART DISEASE

As with diabetes, doctors have long known that some families have more members with kidney disease than others. Kidney disease is an inherited risk factor, and heart disease is the most common cause of death among people who have kidney disease. What's the connection? When the heart is no longer pumping efficiently, it becomes congested with blood, causing pressure to build up in the main vein connected to the kidneys and leading to blood congestion in the kidneys too. The kidneys also suffer from the reduced supply of oxygenated blood.

When the kidneys become impaired, the hormone system, which regulates blood pressure, goes into overdrive in an attempt to increase blood supply to the kidneys. The heart then has to pump against higher pressure in the arteries and eventually suffers from the increase in workload.

If you have diabetes and have a brother, sister, or parent with diabetic kidney disease, the chance that you will develop kidney disease is higher. Genes might be part of the reason that African American, Hispanic, Pacific Islander, Native American, and Native Alaskan people have higher risks. If you have diabetes but do not have a relative with diabetic kidney disease, you have a lower chance of developing that condition over the course of your lifetime.

As with diabetes, researchers are pursuing how genes affect kidney disease and its correlation with heart disease, and for one researcher the quest is personal. "My grandfather had hypertension for 45 years," says Dr. Sun Woo Kang, a South Korean–born nephrologist and researcher with a fellowship from the National Kidney Foundation. "My father has had diabetes and hypertension for 25 years. He also had heart bypass surgery. Then, it was recently discovered that I had certain precursors for cardiovascular or kidney disease similar to my father, and my father's father. I became even more interested in human genetics as it relates to cardiovascular disease and kidney disease," he said in an interview published on the National Kidney Foundation's website. Kang's study—one of many looking at the genetic connection between chronic kidney disease and chronic heart disease—is currently underway at the Center for Human Genetics and Genomics at the University of California, San Diego.

10

DIET

When I opened my cardiology practice more than sixty years ago, the concept of dieting was simple: to stay fit, eat less. There was little thought as to whether what you ate might actually be promoting heart disease. Since then, I've watched diet fads come and go—and sometimes come back again.

In the 1970s the Scarsdale diet was all the rage. It had a simple premise: all one had to do to stay fit was eat one thousand calories or less, no matter one's body size, gender, or level of activity. This one-size-fits-all plan quickly lost favor as consumers found that it was easier said than done.

The Pritikin diet defined thinking about weight loss in the 1980s. It advocated a low-fat, high-fiber diet. Its emphasis on limiting intake of red meat and processed food was a precursor to the vegetarian diets that would become popular two generations later. But devotees tired of its limited food choices and a feeling of constant hunger.

In the 1990s the Atkins diet became the first popular high-protein, high-fat, low-carb diet. The whole idea behind the diet was that excessive body fat was caused by consuming not only fatty foods but also foods consisting of carbohydrates and particularly simple carbs. Americans were by then no doubt consuming excessive amounts of food loaded with simple carbohydrates like sugary soft drinks, candy, cakes, and food products manufactured with fructose. But again, many consumers found that the diet often did not help them maintain weight loss over the long term. And the simple truth of the matter is that some simple carbohydrates, such as fresh fruits and vegetables, are good for you (although they still need to be monitored for total caloric intake).

A few years later the Zone diet captured the public's attention. Like the Atkins diet, it emphasized high protein and low carbs, and fat intake was carefully monitored and controlled. Its signature directive was that followers had to eat five times a day in order to maintain their proper glycemic index. The diet fell out of favor as consumers found it difficult to stick to the multiple daily meals.

Remember the South Beach diet of the early 2000s? The foundational theory behind this diet was classifying carbohydrates as good or bad. It was the Zone diet but without the five-meal requirement and no calorie restriction. To its credit, distinguishing between simple and complex carbohydrates made sense.

And who can forget the Paleo "caveman" diet, based on the 1890s writing of Dr. John Harvey Kellogg, who posited that the primitive diet of humans, while they were still primarily hunter-gatherers, was superior to the diet that emerged after the advent of agriculture. (There's no little irony here that Kellogg also invented the modern-day breakfast cereal. Yep, that Kellogg.) In 2013 the Paleo diet was the most popular among Google searches, as followers adhered to a diet of lean meats, fish, fruits, vegetables, nuts, and seeds and avoided all grains, potatoes, legumes, salt, sugar, dairy, and processed foods.

Now, in 2020, where are we when it comes to dieting? The cold harsh reality is that while all these diets worked for some people at least some of the time, for most people they did not. Two-thirds of Americans today are either overweight or obese, and childhood obesity has tripled in the past three decades.

Which brings me to my patient Nathan. A boyish-looking thirty-six-year-old, he nevertheless was definitely on the older end of the Millennial Generation. At five feet, ten inches tall and weighing 240 pounds, Nathan was definitely overweight, and in pursuit of a slimmer self, he had tried all the diets I just mentioned. No kidding.

"But Nathan, you weren't even born when some of these diets were popular. How did you even find them?" I asked him.

"What can I say, Doc? I'm a great researcher. I even found some of the diet books in a box in my parents' basement," he said.

Nathan worked in video game development for a large company in Los Angeles's "Silicon Beach"—the area formerly known as Playa Vista (just south of Marina del Rey) that has become the high-tech nexus for the city. A typical day for him was sitting in front of a computer screen doing whatever video game developers do. He rarely exercised. In fact, during the day he rarely moved. His sedentary lifestyle was exacerbated by his frat-boy diet, which consisted of mainly fast or frozen foods, and his blood panel revealed excessive amounts of sodium and dangerously high levels of LDL cholesterol. He was a prime candidate for silent heart disease.

"Maybe you should create a diet video game?" I mused.

"Funny, Doc. For some reason, I don't think that would ever fly with the higher-ups," he said.

"But seriously, to find the secret to a healthy diet, you have to go much further back than thirty, forty, or fifty years. We have to go back to ancient Greece," I told him.

"Now you've got my attention."

In fact, the notion of a diet harkens back to the ancient Greek word *diata*, which referred to a philosophy of self-control and eating in moderation. The Greeks and Romans understood that food and exercise influenced fitness and weight. The Christians later reinterpreted this self-control as asceticism, with a denial of worldly pleasures as the only true pathway to the elevation of the soul. Gluttony was one of the cardinal sins of thirteenth-century Christendom, right up there with greed, wrath, sloth, and lust.

Not until the 1940s would we have the first inkling of a connection between diet and heart health. As noted earlier in the book, medical scientists began to seriously look at heart disease as a national health epidemic when the number of deaths attributed to the condition in the United States in one year eclipsed the total number of Americans who died in combat or from combat-related accidents during all of World War II. Seemingly healthy, middle-aged men were dropping dead in the streets of America, and one area the scientists turned their gaze toward in search of clues was diet.

LINK BETWEEN HEART DISEASE AND DIET

One early key piece of research in establishing the correlation between heart health and diet was the Seven Countries Study led by Ancel Keys, an American physiologist who specialized in researching the impact of diet on health. He launched the Seven Countries Study in 1958, after exploratory research on the relationship between dietary patterns and the prevalence of coronary heart disease in Greece, Italy, Spain, South Africa, Japan, and Finland.

There were two key findings: (1) high levels of cholesterol in blood serum were associated with a high risk of coronary heart disease mortality, and (2) a Mediterranean-style diet was consistently associated with lower cardiovascular risk by as much as 39 percent. Subsequent research, including the famed Framingham Heart Study in the United States a few years later, confirmed as much. However, for the next twenty years or so, we barely heard a peep about the Mediterranean diet, despite the seemingly convincing evidence of its efficacy in fighting coronary artery heart disease. For reasons that perhaps harken back to America's Puritan beginnings, doctors and patients—even the American Heart Association (AHA)—alike became laser-focused on fat as bad, no matter that the Mediterranean diet rejected that myopic view. (There's that venal sin of gluttony rearing its ugly head again.)

Not until 1977 did the AHA finally begin adopting recommendations that mimicked the Mediterranean diet with its publication of "Dietary Goals in the United States"—the first comprehensive statement by any branch of government on heart disease risk factors in the American diet. It advised that "too much fat, too much sugar or salt in a diet could be directly linked to heart disease, and stroke . . . and told Americans to eat more fruits, vegetables, whole grains, poultry, and fish."

Just a few years later, AHA changed gears again and returned to an emphasis on controlling dietary fat in a consensus report titled "Lowering Blood Cholesterol to Prevent Heart Disease," which was endorsed by the American Medical Association and the National Heart, Lung, and Blood Institute. Although some scientists and physicians remained unconvinced by the data, nevertheless, the low-fat contingency won the day, and the Mediterranean diet once again fell into obscurity.

"So, Nathan, you've become somewhat of a diet expert. Have you heard of the Mediterranean diet?"

"Um, is that what they eat in Italy? I love lasagna, by the way."

WHAT IS THE MEDITERRANEAN DIET?

The Mediterranean diet really isn't just one diet but rather an umbrella term for many culinary traditions of the countries that border the Mediterranean Sea. To Nathan's point, yes, Italian food falls under the umbrella, but so do the diverse cuisines of Spain, Turkey, Israel, Morocco, and Lebanon. Despite their flavorful difference, they share a common foundation. Their dishes are typically low in red meat, sugar, and saturated fats and high in fresh vegetables, fruit, seafood, nuts, legumes, and whole grains.

While France is on the Mediterranean Sea, the primary fat in its sophisticated cuisine is animal-based, mainly butter and cream. On the other hand, the fat primarily used in the Mediterranean diet is olive oil. In fact, the countries of the Mediterranean diet are sometimes referred to as the olive-growing region of the world. The foods in this region are nutrient rich and are packed with minerals, protein, whole grains, and other nutrients but are lower in calories than the typical American diet. Seasoning leans toward spices rather than salt.

There isn't an emphasis on less fat per se but rather on nutrient-dense whole foods. Indeed, some foods that are "fatty" are essential to a Mediterranean diet. Olive oil supplies monounsaturated fatty acid, and the fish, nuts, and whole grains supply omega-3 and omega-6 fatty acids. Thus, there is ample supply of the essential fatty acids. That said, in the Mediterranean diet, fat makes up only about 30 percent of total calories. The consumption of meat and dairy products high in saturated fats is minimal, and the overall intake of saturated fat is low, typically less than 10 percent of total calories.

Related to the Mediterranean diet is the Dietary Approaches to Stop Hypertension (DASH) diet, which mimics the same kinds of foods but also places special emphasis on reducing salt. Followers begin capping sodium at twenty-three hundred milligrams a day, eventually lowering their daily intake to about fifteen hundred milligrams.

NEW RESEARCH AND THE BENEFITS OF EATING MEDITERRANEAN

Now, we come full circle. As I write, a new study was released in August 2019 confirming the original findings of the Seven Countries Study. Released by none other than the American Heart Association, the study concludes that eating mostly plant-based foods and fewer animal-based foods may be linked to better heart health and a lower risk of dying from a heart attack, stroke, or other cardiovascular disease.

Lead researcher Casey M. Rebholz, PhD, assistant professor of epidemiology at the Johns Hopkins Bloomberg School of Public Health, in

Baltimore, Maryland, and her team reviewed a database of food intake information from more than ten thousand middle-aged U.S. adults who were monitored from 1987 through 2016 and did not have cardiovascular disease at the start of the study. They then categorized the participants' eating patterns by the proportion of plant-based foods they ate versus animal-based foods.

People who ate the most plant-based foods overall had the following:

- 16 percent lower risk of having a cardiovascular disease such as heart attack, stroke, heart failure, and other conditions
- 32 percent lower risk of dying from a cardiovascular disease
- 25 percent lower risk of dying from any cause compared to those who ate the least amount of plant-based foods

"Our findings underscore [that] . . . to reduce cardiovascular disease risk people should eat more vegetables, nuts, whole grains, fruits, legumes and fewer animal-based foods. These findings are pretty consistent with previous findings about other dietary patterns, including the DASH diet, which emphasize the same food items," Rebholz said. And I might add, the Mediterranean diet.

THE RISE OF VEGETARIANISM

I would be remiss in our discussion of heart-healthy diets if I didn't discuss vegetarianism. Like the Mediterranean diet, it takes many forms. Some vegetarians eat no animal protein (vegans), others eat dairy products (lacto-ovo vegetarians), and still others eat fish (pescatarians). It might be better to think of these diets as "pro-vegetarian" because they all emphasize to varying degrees a diet based on fresh fruits and vegetables, nuts, whole grains, and legumes—like the Mediterranean diet.

The benefits of a pro-vegetarian diet were confirmed in a study whose findings were published in April 2019 in the *Journal of the American College of Cardiology*. Dr. Kyla Lara, a cardiology fellow at the Mayo Clinic in Rochester, Minnesota, and her colleagues examined the associations between five major dietary patterns and the risk of heart failure among people without any known history of heart disease. Namely, they looked at the dietary patterns among 16,068 black and white people who were forty-five years old, on average. The participants answered a 150-item survey, which included 107 food items. The researchers grouped the foods into dietary patterns:

- "Convenience" diets, which consisted of meat-heavy dishes, pasta, pizza, and fast food
- "Plant-based" diets, consisting mainly of vegetables, fruit, beans, and fish
- "Southern" diets, which comprised a significant amount of fried foods, processed meat, eggs, added fats, and sugary drinks
- "Alcohol/salad" diets, which included lots of wine, liquor, beer, leafy greens, and salad dressing

Lara and her team followed the participants for 8.7 years on average. Overall, the researchers found that adhering to the southern diet increased the risk of hospitalization due to heart failure by 72 percent, while sticking to a diet rich in fruits, vegetables, and fish can slash heart failure risk by 40 percent.

A similar finding by another study was essentially that you don't have to eat strictly vegetarian to reap the benefits of a Mediterranean-style diet. A team from Erasmus University Medical Center, based in Rotterdam, the Netherlands, examined long-term health information collected as part of the Rotterdam study. The data included 9,641 adults with an average age of sixty-two years who took part in this ongoing population-based study. In particular, the researchers were interested in the participants' diet, body mass index (BMI), waist circumference, weight in relation to height (fat mass index), and body fat percentage.

The participants received points for eating nuts, fruits, and vegetables and lost points for eating meat, dairy, and fish. So the higher individuals' scores, the more closely they adhered to a plant-based diet. The team found that people with the highest scores on the index were more likely to have a lower BMI over the long term.

Lead study author Zhangling Chen concluded, "Eating a plant-based diet to protect against obesity does not require a radical change in diet or a total elimination of meat or animal products. Instead, it can be achieved in various ways, such as moderate reduction of red meat consumption or eating a few more vegetables. This supports current recommendations to shift to diets rich in plant foods with low consumption of animal foods."

NATHAN GOES MEDITERRANEAN

"Wow. So, switching to a plant-based diet will turn my health around, eh, Doc? You know, I just got turned on to cauliflower cheese pizza. And french fries are vegetarian, too, right?" said Nathan.

"Now, hold on. The fact that we're reducing the animal protein in your diet isn't a license for you to binge on other kinds of bad food. There's very little nutritional value in either cauliflower cheese pizza or French fries, and they're probably loaded with salt," I said.

"You mean I'll be chained to broccoli and arugula for the rest of my life?"

"Not exclusively, but they will be part of your new Mediterranean diet, filled with fresh fruits and vegetables and low in salt, sugar, and processed foods, including sugary soft drinks and those packaged baked goods containing trans fats. Your days of fast and frozen food are gone. Instead, you're eating fresh fish at least twice a week, especially fish high in omega-3 fatty acids like tuna and salmon. If you choose to eat meat, look for the leanest cuts available and prepare them in healthy and delicious ways. And you'll select fiber-rich whole grains for most grain servings."

I continued, "You said you like Italian food, right? How about Spanish, Turkish, or Lebanese? If you are not familiar with these cuisines, well, Nathan, you're about to experience a whole new world of food."

"Hmmm. The Mediterranean diet video game. An army of fruits, nuts, and legumes combats the dark forces of red meat, sugar, and salt. Throw in some wizards and ogres, and we might have a hit, Doc!"

"And don't forget the brass ring is improved cardiovascular health," I chimed in.

"Yeah, I'll get the marketing team to work on that last part."

(There are scores of cookbooks for the Mediterranean diet available online or at your local bookstore. For a list of foods and suggested meals on the Mediterranean diet that I recommended for Nathan, visit the Eating Well website at http://www.eatingwell.com/article/291946/30 -day-mediterranean-diet-meal-plan-1200-calories.)

11

SEDENTARY LIFESTYLE

In the last chapter, we learned how the medical profession's and the public's understanding of how poor diet can be an important risk factor for silent heart disease and coronary heart disease in general has dramatically increased over the last fifty years. The same is true with exercise. When I first began my cardiology practice, any discussion of how activity might influence the development of cardiovascular disease focused on how too much exercise or physical exertion might trigger a heart attack. If you didn't physically exert yourself—at all—then you were minimizing your chance of a heart attack.

How the times are a-changin' (apology to Bob Dylan!). Today, a wide body of research shows that a sedentary lifestyle—in which the majority of your daily routine consists of sitting or sleeping—is not only not alright but downright dangerous. That's not to say that the opposite is necessarily true—that exercise fanatics automatically decrease their risk of coronary heart disease. (More on this later in the chapter.) But there's little doubt that moderate activity multiple times per day does significantly reduce your risk of heart disease.

Even if your weight is normal and you exercise intensely once or twice a week, if the majority of your waking hours on all the other days is spent sitting, you're still living the kind of sedentary lifestyle that the American Heart Association (AHA) is ringing alarm bells about. This is from a recent "scientific advisory" from the AHA, which issues such reports on important issues in order to inform physicians: "There is now a substantial body of prospective data on associations of sedentary behavior with risk of developing cardiovascular disease as well as with overall mortality. Several (mainly cross-sectional) studies have also found significant associations of sedentary time (deleterious) and breaks from sedentary time (protective) with risk biomarkers."

In short, inactivity equals death. Dramatic? Yes, but as we dig deeper into the science behind these latest findings, we now understand that the human body is meant to move. Inactivity not only fails to maximize the body's health potential but, even more importantly, can actually promote a whole cascade of illnesses, including silent heart disease.

A MOVING STATEMENT

In our last chapter, you met my patient Nathan, the thirty-six-year-old, overweight video game programmer. Part of the reason for his high-risk profile for coronary heart disease was his diet. We solved that problem by switching him from a diet consisting largely of fast and frozen foods to a healthful Mediterranean diet, which emphasized fresh fruits and vegetables, fresh fish, whole grains, and olive oil. But diet was only part of Nathan's health problem, the other being his sedentary lifestyle.

You know, being a Beverly Hills cardiologist, I've run into my share of entertainment industry professionals—actors, editors, producers, directors, and so forth—and actually have visited some of them at their work. The public perception of a movie set is an intense beehive of activity. Lights, camera, action!—right? Indeed, there is a certain creative energy that's buzzing all around on a TV or movie set, but the reality is that there's a good deal of just sitting around and waiting—for both the cast and the crew. For the most part, it's sedentary.

With video games, where even the set is virtual, not to mention the cast, the level of inactivity reaches new heights. Like most professionals in his industry, Nathan sits in front of a computer monitor during his working day, with typing on his keyboard or moving his computer mouse the only regular activity that he engages in.

"Aren't you proud of me, Doc? I've lost twenty-five pounds on the Mediterranean diet and I'm feeling and looking better than ever," said Nathan on a recent visit.

"Yes, congratulations. The results are impressive. But we've only just begun," I said.

"Wait! I thought the Mediterranean diet was the end game?"

"Let me ask you this, Nathan. How often do you exercise?

"Ah, I got you there, Doc. I am a weekend warrior to the ninja degree. I mean, I go to the gym either on Saturday or Sunday for at least two hours, sometimes three hours. Weights, cycling, the whole nine yards," he said proudly.

"And otherwise during the week, how often are you active?"

"Not much, but, you see, I bank all my good physical activity on the weekends so I can just cruise through the week." he said.

"Unfortunately, it doesn't work that way. Maintaining good cardio health means being active on a daily basis," I advised. "The good news is just a little activity goes a long way."

BMI ISN'T EVERYTHING

A fairly recent innovation in the measurement of good health has been the body mass index (BMI). This value, derived from the weight of the person cross-referenced with his or her height, is a convenient rule of thumb used to broadly categorize a person as underweight, normal weight, overweight, or obese, based on tissue mass (muscle, fat, and bone) and height. So far, so good. However, this weight-to-height ratio can lull people into believing that a "normal" BMI means they're the picture of perfect health.

In reality, BMI is a crude marker of sedentary behavior. It doesn't predict whether a person is engaging in enough daily activity to sustain a heart-healthy lifestyle. In a study published in 2019 in the *American Journal of Cardiology*, researchers at the University of Florida in Gainesville found that a lifestyle characterized by daily physical inactivity can put healthy-weight adults at the same risk for cardiovascular disease as adults who are overweight. "Our study demonstrates that a sedentary lifestyle counters the benefit of being at a normal weight when it comes to heart disease risk," said lead investigator Arch G. Mainous III, PhD, in an interview published in *Cath Lab Digest*. "Achieving a body mass index, or BMI, in the normal range shouldn't give people a false sense of confidence they're in good health. If you're not exercising, you're not doing enough."

Researchers examined participants' fat in the gut region as well as waist circumference. In addition, they calculated participants'

Atherosclerotic Cardiovascular Disease (ASCVD) risk score, based on an algorithm devised by the American College of Cardiology and the American Heart Association. The ASCVD risk score uses weighted variables, including age, sex, race/ethnicity, smoking status, diabetes status, cholesterol level, blood pressure, and blood pressure medication status, to determine individuals' risk of having a heart attack or stroke within the next ten years. A score of 7.5 percent or higher is considered high risk.

What did the research find? Two things that are counterintuitive and actually quite shocking:

- The rate of high ASCVD risk score among overweight people was similar to the rate among people who had a normal BMI but had indicators of a sedentary lifestyle.
- 30 percent of U.S. adults of normal weight are at increased risk of heart attack or stroke.

The test subjects in the Gainesville study had higher levels of belly fat, shortness of breath upon exertion, unhealthy waist circumference, or less than recommended levels of physical activity, but again their weight scale and their BMI measurement indicated a clean bill of health.

As we learned earlier, silent heart disease is a special kind of coronary heart disease in that it's asymptomatic. Thus, patients who are seemingly healthy based on their BMI might think that they have a very low risk of silent heart disease when, in fact, they might have a whole range of factors increasing their risk of heart disease . . . including a sedentary lifestyle.

Let's dig a little deeper into the study. The investigators analyzed data from the National Health and Nutrition Examination Survey, a nationally representative study that collects data from a combination of interviews, physical examinations, and laboratory tests. The study focuses on participants ages forty to seventy-nine with no previous diagnosis of coronary heart disease, stroke, or heart attack.

"We have traditionally thought that people with a normal BMI are healthy and at low risk for heart disease, but increasingly we are finding that how much you weigh is not necessarily a measure of good health," said Mainous, the lead researcher. "Sedentary lifestyle markers may play a better role in predicting cardiovascular disease risk."

Exactly!

A WIDENING PROBLEM

According to the American Heart Association, sedentary jobs have increased 83 percent since 1950. Physically active work now makes up less than 20 percent of U.S. jobs, down from roughly half of jobs in 1960.

So what the heck happened to the fitness craze that emerged in the 1980s with the likes of Jane Fonda and aerobics and Jim Fixx and jogging? What happened was that even as average Americans joined in more sports activities than their parents, they were becoming more and more tied to a desk. The advent of computer technology and the Information Age in the 1990s sealed the deal.

The end result was Americans' striving to be more physically active but eventually losing the battle. And as I discussed with my patient Nathan earlier, it's not as if you can bank your physical activity and use its benefits later on in the week. If you're crazy active during the weekends but essentially inactive during the workweek, you're not improving your heart health. To reframe this paradox, sedentary behavior can coexist with high levels of total physical activity.

A large review of studies published in 2015 in the *Annals of Internal Medicine* found that even after adjusting for physical activity, sitting for long periods was associated with worse health outcomes, including heart disease, but also type 2 diabetes, which, as we discussed in Chapter 9, is also a risk factor for cardiovascular disease.

Historically, research on physical activity focused on the relationship between energy expenditure and health benefits. The resulting physical activity guidelines were largely oriented toward increasing physical activity levels in the population rather than reducing sedentary behavior. To be clear, we have known for millennia that physical activity improves overall health. None other than Hippocrates and Siddhartha sang the praises of exercise. But it was a British epidemiologist, Jeremy N. Morris, who first proved in the 1950s that the opposite was also true—that inactivity or sedentary behavior wasn't benign but was actually bad for you.

Who were the subjects of his study? Employees of the London transport department. Morris had a hunch that prolonged inactivity was an important risk factor for coronary disease, but how could he show it? He happened upon the idea while riding one of London's iconic double-decker buses. He noticed that drivers of the buses sat continually, never moving from their perch behind the wheels. On the other hand, the conductors who took the tickets were constantly on the move, walking up and down the aisles and even up and down the buses' circular staircases. To be precise, the drivers sat for 90 percent of their shifts; the conductors climbed about six hundred stairs each working day.

So, all things considered, here were two sets of test subjects who worked in exactly the same environment, and the only thing that differentiated them was their job description. If there was a discrepancy in the risk of cardiovascular disease between the active and inactive in their daily work routine, it should reveal itself here on London's buses.

Morris studied thirty-one thousand employees aged thirty-five to sixty-four during two years from 1949 to 1950. So, what did he find? The research was conclusive. When compared with conductors, bus drivers had about double the age-adjusted rate of fatal coronary heart disease. This was the first indication that sedentary behavior could markedly increase cardiovascular heart disease risk.

Ever the careful scientist, Morris set out to replicate the study. After all, maybe an unforeseen factor was influencing the results. For example, maybe people with certain body types were more prone to seek jobs with little activity (like driving a bus). The London transport department provided him with the trouser sizes of its workers. His data indicated that while conductors' waistbands were smaller, their protection against heart attack could not be explained by a lean body type. The conductors had a lower risk of heart attack whether they were slim, average size, or portly.

Then, to corroborate his findings further, Morris turned his inquisitive mind toward London's postal workers. He compared those who delivered the mail by walking or riding a bicycle with the window clerks at the post office and the telephone operators. And the results? (Drum roll, please.) The constantly on the move deliverers had a far lower risk of heart attack than their sedentary counterparts, the clerks and operators.

Morris would go on to show in subsequent studies that inactivity was also bad for those who had already had a heart attack. Prior to his research, heart attack victims were prescribed a regimen of as little physical exertion as possible. His continuing research showed the opposite was warranted: exercise reduced the risk of heart attack. (Morris, who followed his own prescriptive advice about staying active on a daily basis, lived until he was 99.5 years old.)

THE TV FACTOR

Now, you may ask, if inactivity is bad, are some kinds worse than others? As turns out, the answer is yes, according to the latest research.

An analysis of data from several thousand US participants aged fifty to seventy-one years in a study conducted by the National Institutes of Health and the AARP showed that the risk of cardiovascular disease rose progressively in lockstep with time spent watching television or videos. Participants' time spent watching television or videos was assessed with the question "During a typical 24-h period over the past 12 months, how much time did you spend watching television or videos?" Among participants who watched one hour versus seven hours of television or videos per day, the heavy TV watchers had almost double the incidence of coronary heart disease.

These findings were validated in a subsequent study, published in 2019 in the *Journal of the American Heart Association*, which focused on binge TV watching compared to the effects of occupational sitting, such as at desk jobs. Over eight years researchers studied 3,592 adults enrolled in the Jackson Heart Study, a large, ongoing, community-based study following adults living in Jackson, Mississippi. With all other factors (e.g., age, occupation, gender) considered, those who watched the most television in their hours of inactivity had disproportionately higher rates of heart disease and stroke and faced a greater risk of cardiovascular disease at all ages of life. Even sustained and regular exercise proved not to offset the results.

You can almost hear the collective groan from Hollywood TV executives that, once again, they've been made the scapegoats for society's ills. TV watching is blamed for everything from mental illness to gun violence; why not add to the list increased risk of coronary heart disease?

It turns out, however, there's a simple explanation. According to the study's lead researcher, Jeanette Garcia, PhD, a professor of kinesiology and physical therapy at the University of Central Florida in Orlando,

"TV watching may be associated with heart health risks more than sitting at work [because] TV watching occurs at the end of the day where individuals may consume their biggest meal, and people may be completely sedentary with hours of uninterrupted sitting until they go to bed. Eating a large meal and then sitting hours at a time could be a very harmful combination." Snacking may also be an issue and, unfortunately, individuals typically are not snacking on fresh fruits and vegetables, but rather potato chips or other sweet or salty, high-calorie foods. At a desk job, workers are often getting up, going to a copy machine, talking with a colleague, going to a meeting or to the break room. It's not hours of uninterrupted sitting.

EXERCISE DOSING

So, if some sedentary behavior is worse than other kinds, how about exercise? Is some better in preventing cardiovascular heart disease?

There continues to be considerable controversy about the optimal dose of physical activity. However, substantial evidence suggests that any level of physical exercise and activity is better than none. Current federal guidelines call for a minimum of 150 minutes per week of moderate aerobic physical activity or 75 minutes per week of vigorous physical activity. The majority of Americans do not meet these guidelines, with only 10 percent meeting this minimum recommended level of activity.

Runners have the best results, according to studies. However, interesting findings emerge when we assess running dosing by dividing runners into quintiles of exercise volumes, such as miles per week, times per week, and minutes per week. Research shows that those who run less than six miles per week, one to two times per week, had the same benefits in preventing coronary heart disease as those who ran much more and more often.

There's even some evidence that those who ran the most actually decreased the effects of their exercise in preventing cardiovascular disease. In other words, even though moderate levels of exercise have been found to be consistently associated with a reduction in coronary disease risk, there is evidence to suggest that continuously high levels of exercise (e.g., marathon running) could have detrimental effects on cardiovascular health.

MECHANISM OF ACTIVITY VERSUS INACTIVITY

Alright, so excessive and regular inactivity is bad. But what is the physiological mechanism by which exercise imparts it remarkable benefits to cardiovascular health and conversely causes sustained inactivity to be so perilous?

The short answer is that we don't know for sure. However, many studies have tested whether regular engagement in physical activity may lower the risk of cardiovascular disease by affecting the levels of circulating lipoproteins. These studies have found that endurance training is associated with elevated levels of circulating high-density lipoprotein (HDL) and, to a lesser extent, a reduction in triglyceride levels—both changes that can reduce the risk of coronary heart disease.

Also, we know that blood flow increases in a standing versus a sitting position and is further increased during physical activity in response to increased oxygen requirements in muscle. There are clearly physiological changes that occur when physically active individuals become inactive. Reduced insulin sensitivity is found during prolonged sedentary behavior that can be mitigated with short bouts of physical activity.

RECOMMENDATIONS

Despite the extensive body of knowledge documenting the unequivocal health benefits of exercise, a vast majority of Americans do not engage in sufficient physical activity. Nonetheless, mortality risk reduction appears with even small bouts of daily exercise and peaks at fifty to sixty minutes of vigorous exercise each day.

However, the question remains as to how much exercise is optimal for cardiovascular health benefit. Studies in endurance runners show that the frequency of adverse cardiovascular events in marathoners is equivalent to that in a population with established coronary heart disease, suggesting that too much exercise may be detrimental. An upper limit for the cardiovascular benefits of exercise is further supported by a recent study showing that individuals who completed at least twenty-five marathons over a period of twenty-five years had higher than expected levels of coronary artery calcification (CAC) and calcified coronary plaque volume compared with sedentary individuals. (CAC scoring, also called a coronary calcium scan, is a test that measures the amount of calcium in the walls of the heart's arteries. A coronary calcium scan is one way to estimate someone's risk of developing heart disease or having a heart attack or stroke.)

Another recent investigation also showed that individuals who maintain very high levels of physical activity (three times recommended levels) have higher odds of developing CAC, particularly white males. In contrast, other studies report greater plaque stability due to calcification in exercisers, indicating that with higher levels of physical activity, plaque quality may be favorably impacted to lower the risk of cardiovascular events, despite a higher incidence of plaques and abnormal CAC scores.

An immediate result of a change from a highly physical active state to a highly sedentary state is a reduction in muscle and systemic insulin sensitivity, and if the resulting energy imbalance is sustained, adipose or fat tissue will expand. The consequences of energy surplus, adiposity, and insulin resistance for inflammation and cardiovascular disease risk have been well established. A decrease in insulin sensitivity that results from becoming sedentary can occur independent of increased adiposity or energy surplus.

To summarize, researchers believe there is a sweet spot between enough and too much exercise. It appears that both too little activity and too much activity can trigger physiological inflammation, which is in and of itself a well-known risk factor for cardiovascular disease.

REALITY CHECK

For most of us, running twenty-five marathons is a distant likelihood, and so exercising too much shouldn't be a concern for 90 percent of adult Americans. But here's the best part: even a nominal increase in activity—for example, only sitting five hours instead of ten—results in a decreased risk of fatal and nonfatal coronary heart disease.

For those looking to increase to an optimum activity level, the Centers for Disease Control and Prevention has published physical activity guidelines, which recommend at least 150 minutes of moderate-intensity exercise a week for adults. Exercise should include a combination of aerobic activity and strength training. I recommended such an activity regimen for my patient Nathan.

"Continue Mediterranean diet, check. Two-plus hours of moderate exercise *but* spread out throughout the week. Anything else, Doc?" said Nathan.

"Yes, get up and walk around," I said.

"You mean now?"

"No, at work. Every hour, I want you to leave whatever virtual world you're creating and reconnect with reality—get up from your desk and go get a glass of water, say hi to a colleague, stretch and touch your toes. Do you think your digital menagerie of creatures can let you be away for that long? Remember, there's a great deal of benefit to light activity during the day but only if you do it throughout the day."

"Got it. The body—at least the human body—is designed to keep moving."

12

OBESITY

One of the most disheartening aspects of my sixty-year career in cardiology has been witnessing a steady decline in the rate of heart disease in America, only to have victory snatched by the jaws of defeat. Yes, heart disease affects one in four Americans, and for almost a century now it has remained the leading cause of death in the United States. But in the mid-1970s, after a sixty-year gradual increase as the U.S. population aged, there was a significant downtick in the frequency of cardiovascular heart disease and related stroke mortality rates.

By 2000, mortality rates from heart disease had declined to about one-third their 1960s baseline. From 2006 to 2016, the annual death rate attributable to coronary heart disease declined by 31.8 percent, and the actual number of deaths declined 14.6 percent.

That remarkable progress in battling the leading killer of Americans was fueled by both improved treatment and prevention. The huge and costly public information campaigns about the dangers of cigarette smoking and about lowering cholesterol through a change to a more healthful diet, the widespread use of statin and other medications to lower cholesterol, and improvements in preventing and treating hypertension were paying off. Again, the war against heart disease was by no means over, but after four decades of lowering its rate, heart disease seemed to be on the run, and the day when it was no longer the leading cause of death in America was actually in sight.

Then came the bad news in May 2019. In an article published in the *Journal of the American College of Cardiology*, a comprehensive study conducted by Northwestern University, found death rates due to heart failure were now increasing and, even worse, actually had been increasing since 2012.

The study used data from the National Health and Nutrition Examination Survey, a program of studies conducted by the Centers for Disease Control and Prevention (CDC) designed to assess the health and nutritional status of adults and children in the United States. The survey is unique in that it combines interviews and physical examinations and provides a snapshot of the overall health of the nation. In short, the data and its conclusions were definitive.

As lead researcher Dr. Sadiya Khan, assistant professor of medicine at Northwestern University's Feinberg School of Medicine and a Northwestern cardiologist, noted in the published article, the rise in deaths came despite significant advances in medical and surgical treatments for heart failure in the past decade. The cause of this discouraging reversal in what had been steady progress for more than forty years? In a word, obesity, or to be more precise, the nation's current obesity epidemic.

I don't use the word "epidemic" lightly, but there is no other way to describe the dramatic increase in rates of obesity in the United States, which, as it turns out, have paralleled an increased rate of heart failure. According to the latest statistics from the CDC, 39.6 percent of adults and 18.5 percent of children ages two to nineteen are obese in America. Let's pause for a moment and reflect on those numbers. If you were to walk into any public venue in the United States today—a bank, a restaurant, a house of worship, an airport—on average four out of ten adults there would be clinically obese, and nearly one out of five children would qualify as obese as well. Those are chilling statistics.

To be perfectly honest, it's not like my colleagues in cardiology didn't notice that patients were, well, getting larger—much larger—over the last twenty years. In fact, the origins of the obesity epidemic can be traced all the way back to 1962, when the first uptick in obesity rates were documented; since then, the obesity rate has increased steadily.

"The success of the last three decades in improving heart disease death rates is now being reversed, and it is likely due to the obesity and diabetes epidemics," said Khan. "We focused on patients with heart failure because they have the highest mortality related to cardiovascular death. They have a prognosis similar to metastatic lung cancer."

In other words, while the study doesn't document it, it's likely that other kinds of coronary heart conditions like silent heart disease have also increased.

An estimated 6 million adults in the United States have heart failure. What exactly is meant by heart failure? Simply put, heart failure is when the heart muscle doesn't function properly in its squeezing and/or relaxing functions. This causes symptoms like shortness of breath and swelling. When the heart can't adequately squeeze to pump blood, it's called "heart failure with usually reduced ejection fraction"; when the heart can't relax, it is called "heart failure with preserved ejection fraction." About 50 percent of individuals diagnosed with heart failure (of either kind) will die within the next five years.

"Given the aging population and the obesity and diabetes epidemics, which are major risk factors for heart failure, it is likely that this trend will continue to worsen," said Khan.

Recent data show that the average life expectancy in the United States is also declining, which underscores Khan's contention that cardiovascular death related to heart failure may be a significant contributor to this change.

OBESITY EPIDEMIC CAUSES

So, if the obesity is, pardon the pun, at the heart of the increase in fatal coronary heart disease, what caused the obesity epidemic? That is the $64 billion question, which is the estimated annual cost to the U.S. economy in lost productivity because of the obesity epidemic. Then you can add another whopping $147 billion in medical costs related to obesity treatment.

The challenge in the treatment and prevention of obesity is that it's a complex health issue to address. Obesity results from a combination of causes and contributing factors, including diet (notably, the widespread availability and popularity of fast and processed foods over the last five decades), a sedentary lifestyle, and individual behaviors. There's even a genetic component, although the last third of the twentieth century was the first in the history of humans in which obesity became a widespread phenomenon, so it's likely that "nurture" rather than "nature" is more important in the rise of obesity. It's the perfect storm of medical conditions.

However, some well-respected medical researchers believe that, all things considered, something else beyond an increase in sedentary lifestyle and fast foods may be the primary culprit—something far more sinister. In a fascinating book, *The Obesogen Effect*, Dr. Bruce Blumberg, PhD, posits that the obesity epidemic is not the result of too many cheeseburgers or not enough exercise. Rather, Americans' growing waistlines are due to chemical agents found in an array of household goods, from food containers to cleaning and personal care products, which disrupt our hormonal systems. Even worse, his research shows that the effects of these "obesogens" can interfere with the expression of our genes and thereby get passed on from generation to generation.

HOW OBESITY CHANGES THE HEART

It was previously thought that while being overweight might prevent you from achieving maximum health, it was relatively unimportant as a risk factor in coronary heart disease. Now we realize that obesity in and of itself is a major risk factor. In fact, obesity alone affects heart health in a multitude of ways, including by actually changing the structure of the heart.

In a groundbreaking study published in 2019 in the *European Heart Journal*, researchers for the first time found evidence that excess weight and body fat cause a range of heart and blood vessel diseases, rather than just being associated with them. In particular, the study showed that as body mass index (BMI) and fat mass increase, so does the risk of aortic valve stenosis, a condition in which the heart valve controlling the flow of blood from the heart to the body's largest blood vessel, the aorta, narrows and fails to open fully. Blood can back up in other parts of the heart and sometimes the lungs. This can lead to shortness of breath, tiredness, fainting, chest pain, and an irregular heartbeat. While the greatest danger was for aortic valve stenosis (46 percent increased risk), the study found those who were clinically obese were also at a high risk for ischemic stroke, transient ischemic attack, atrial fibrillation, heart failure, and peripheral artery disease.

This was the first heart disease study to use a fascinating new research technique called Mendelian randomization. This technique uses genetic variants that are already known to be associated with potential risk factors, such as BMI and body fat, as indirect indicators of, or "proxies" for, these risk factors. This enables researchers to discover whether the risk factor is the cause of the disease (rather than the other way around) and reduces bias in results because genetic variants are determined at conception and cannot be affected by subsequent external or environmental factors or by the development of disease.

The researchers, led by Susanna Larsson, associate professor and senior researcher at the Karolinska Institute, Stockholm, Sweden, studied ninety-six genetic variants associated with BMI and body fat mass to estimate their effect on fourteen cardiovascular diseases in 367,703 participants of white British descent in UK Biobank, a UK-based national and international resource containing data on five hundred thousand people, aged forty to sixty-nine years. Larsson said, "The causal association between BMI and fat mass and several heart and blood vessel diseases, in particular aortic valve stenosis, was unknown. We found that higher BMI and fat mass are associated with an increased risk of aortic valve stenosis and most other cardiovascular diseases, suggesting that excess body fat is a cause of cardiovascular disease."

There are other ways that obesity physically changes the heart. Being overweight can lead to a buildup of fatty material in the arteries (the blood vessels that carry blood to your organs). If the arteries that carry blood to your heart get damaged and clogged, it can lead to a heart attack. Also, the heavier you are, the more blood you have flowing through your body. The heart has to work harder to pump the extra blood. It stretches, getting bigger and thicker, and the thicker the heart muscle gets, the harder it becomes for it to squeeze and relax with each heartbeat. Gradually, the heart may not be able to keep up with the extra load. You may then have congestive heart failure.

OBESITY CO-OCCURRING DISORDERS

People who have a substance abuse problem oftentimes have what addiction medicine describes as a "co-occurring disorder," or another condition that parallels and contributes to addiction. For example, a person might be addicted to opioid drugs but simultaneously suffer from depression, anxiety, or attention deficit hyperactivity disorder—all common co-occurring disorders of alcohol and drug addiction (which we'll learn more about in the next chapter).

In a sense, obesity has co-occurring disorders, notably high cholesterol, hypertension, and diabetes. As we learned earlier, each of these alone is a risk factor for silent heart disease, but it now appears obesity heightens the risk further.

For example, obese individuals also have a much greater chance of developing diabetes. According to the American Heart Association, at least 68 percent of people aged sixty-five or older with diabetes also have heart disease. Also, obesity can increase the levels of low-density lipoprotein (LDL) cholesterol and triglyceride levels, but it can also lower the good high-density lipoprotein (HDL) cholesterol (which is important in controlling LDL cholesterol). And, finally, as noted earlier, there's a strong correlation between high blood pressure and obesity.

People with severe obesity have a risk of developing heart failure almost four times higher than that of people with an ideal body weight, or the optimal body weight associated with maximum life expectancy (usually as determined by body mass index). Studies also show that the link between obesity and heart failure persists even after accounting for other risk factors. To be clear, if you are obese, you're still at increased risk for heart failure even if you don't have high blood pressure, high cholesterol, or diabetes. As is the case with hypertension or a sedentary lifestyle, this lack of symptoms can make obesity dangerous as a risk factor for silent heart disease.

SYSTEMIC INFLAMMATION

There's still another way obesity increases the risk of heart disease. Obesity contributes to systemic inflammation, which long has been known to have a correlation to heart disease, measured by multiple techniques, including the C-reactive protein blood test.

How exactly does that work? We're not sure yet, but one grand theory—yet to be proven—posits that inflammation in the body is at the roots of many if not most diseases. What we do know today is that an obese person tends to have a disproportionately high volume of a certain kind of adipose tissue called visceral fat. In fact, visceral fat obesity is present in almost 90 percent of obese patients with ischemic heart disease.

Until recently, it was thought that all fat was created equal—a kind of benign tissue that just sat there. Sure, the sheer added weight of excessive fat tissue strained everything in the body, from the heart muscle to knee joints, but its damage seemed to stop there. That is, being forty pounds overweight was like being a normal weight but walking around with a forty-pound weight in your backpack.

However, beginning in the late 1980s and early 1990s, powerful new imaging techniques greatly advanced the understanding of the health risks associated with body fat accumulation. Techniques such as computed tomography and magnetic resonance imaging revealed to medical scientists that there were not one but two different kinds of fat: subcutaneous fat, which sits just below the skin line and often accumulates around the hips, thighs, and buttocks of pear-shaped people, and a more insidious, intra-abdominal fat that surrounds the liver, heart, intestines, and stomach organs and is prominent in apple-shaped people.

Carrying excessive weight around your middle, also called central obesity, can make it harder for your body to use a hormone called insulin, which controls your blood glucose (sugar) levels. This can lead to type 2 diabetes. Having high levels of glucose in your bloodstream damages your arteries and increases your risk of heart and circulatory diseases.

Even worse, visceral fat, far from being benign, functions like a quasi-organ, and may actually produce pro-inflammatory cytokines and adipokines with cardio-depressant and pro-atherosclerotic properties. Visceral fat is typically associated with a westernized diet rich in saturated fats and sugars, which can further contribute to the pro-inflammatory state of patients, particularly since these macronutrients can activate pro-inflammatory pathways.

In the last chapter, we discussed how the body mass index wasn't a particularly good measurement of sedentary lifestyle and, in fact, could mask sedentary behavior as a major risk factor. However, BMI combined with a waist circumference measurement (not necessarily the same as your pants waist size) are a good overall indicator of obesity. Learn how to measure your BMI and waist circumference by following the instructions available on numerous websites, including that of the National Institutes of Health (https://www.nhlbi.nih.gov/health/educational/lose_wt/BMI/bmicalc.htm). Generally speaking, the recommended waist measurements are below 37 inches (94 centimeters) for men and below 31.5 inches (80 centimeters) for women.

CHILDHOOD OBESITY

We'll close this chapter by returning to the new data showing that obesity is a growing problem not only for adults but for children as well. We should all be concerned about a nation of overweight children and adolescents because soon they'll become part of the problem. Obese children and adolescents are more likely to become obese adults with all the risk factors associated with cardiovascular disease (high blood pressure, high cholesterol, type 2 diabetes, and heart attacks).

Also, studies have documented the link between obesity and unhealthy or risky behaviors such as alcohol and tobacco use, premature sexual behavior, inappropriate dieting practices, and physical inactivity. Overweight children and adolescents may experience other health conditions associated with increased weight, including asthma, fatty liver disease, sleep apnea, and type 2 diabetes mellitus.

Finally, obesity puts children at long-term higher risk for chronic conditions such as stroke, musculoskeletal disorders, gallbladder disease, and breast, colon, and kidney cancers.

13

SUBSTANCE ABUSE

Earlier in the book, we learned that heart disease, for nearly one hundred years now, has been the number one killer of Americans and that half of all heart attacks may be "silent"—that is, asymptomatic, or without the chest pain typically associated with heart attacks. Still, great strides have been made over the last six decades in reducing the rate of death from cardiovascular disease through innovations in medications and diagnostics, as well as through you—that is, you the public, who have heeded warnings of how certain behaviors and lifestyle choices can increase the risk of developing silent heart disease and coronary heart disease in general.

In the last chapter, I discussed how much this progress has been undone by the epidemic of obesity. It's a problem that has gradually but steadily grown since the early 1960s, and it had become obvious by the 1990s that obesity posed a major public health risk. The other scourge of the new millennium—drug addiction and particularly the opioid crisis—has followed another trajectory with equally devastating negative effects.

When I was a newly practicing physician in the 1960s, the idea that a huge swath of the American public would abuse illicit drugs—not to mention legally prescribed drugs—to the extent that it became a national health epidemic would have seemed incredible. In fact, the time-released opioid prescription pills that are fueling much of the nation's drug epidemic hadn't even been invented yet. And the two ancient but wildly popular substances with substantial potentials for addiction—nicotine and alcohol—still were not very well understood sixty years ago.

Today, nearly two hundred people die of a drug overdose every day. In 2018, drug overdoses killed more people than guns, car crashes, or HIV/AIDS combined, and in that single year, drug overdose deaths exceeded all U.S. military casualties in the Vietnam and Iraq Wars combined.

Approximately 21 million Americans—almost 8 percent of adolescents and adults—abuse some kind of legal or illegal substance. That number is similar to the number of people who suffer from diabetes and more than 1.5 times the annual prevalence of all cancers combined (14 million).

The abused drugs most associated with cardiovascular disease are opioids, legal (prescription pain medications like oxycodone) and illicit (heroin), and stimulants, notably cocaine and methamphetamine. Collectively these two classes of drugs may increase the risk of vascular and heart disorders by disrupting the balance of certain neurotransmitters, called catecholamines, in the body and brain. This may lead to dose-dependent changes in blood pressure, abnormalities in the rhythms of the heart or blood vessels, and increased blood clotting, arterial plaque formation, and risk of serious events such as heart attacks.

At last the medical profession has begun to realize the effects the opioid epidemic is having on the collective heart health of the nation, and just in time. In addition to the lingering opioid crisis, an old drug scourge that we thought had been left behind for the most part after its heyday in the 1980s, cocaine, is back with us again, but this time with a new and deadly twist.

However, we begin this chapter on substance abuse as a risk factor for silent heart disease and coronary heart disease with a look at two persistent substance abuse problems older than America itself: cigarette smoking and alcohol consumption.

ONE PUFF IS TOO MUCH

When I was growing up, cigarette smoking was very glamorous—seemingly all the golden era movie stars smoked. Later it became very counterculturally cool—a symbol of youthful rebellion. Cigarettes delivered what seemed to be the perfect drug: nicotine. It could pick you up when you were tired or relax you when you were agitated. Sometimes heavy smokers noticed a persistent cough, but what could possibly be wrong with smoking a pack or two a day? OK, maybe cigarettes were not good for you, but too much coffee wasn't either, right?

By the 1980s, the dangers of smoking and its deleterious effect on public health—including cardiovascular disease—had become widely known to just about everybody. The public also became aware of the tobacco industry's efforts to mislead consumers about the health effects of smoking and to manipulate public policy for the short-term interests of the industry. The first successful lawsuits against tobacco companies over smoking-related illness were won at the close of the last century.

We can rejoice that today, because of the cumulative effects of all the educational efforts by many organizations, smoking rates have been cut in half since their apex in the 1960s, when an estimated 42 percent of Americans smoked cigarettes. Today, the proportion is down to just 15 percent. But here's the bad news: that 15 percent, approximately 38 million Americans, somehow did not get the memo that smoking is a leading risk factor for coronary heart disease (not to mention lung cancer) and continue to smoke at least one cigarette per day.

Here's the unique thing about smoking cigarettes—it's absolutely, in the literal sense, dangerous. There's no sliding scale as to how much is maybe OK and how much is really bad. It's all really bad. There are no qualifiers, no equivocations. Medical studies have shown that even light or moderate smoking significantly increases the risk of heart disease.

New research published in 2018 in the *British Medical Journal* revealed that men who smoke one cigarette daily have a 48 percent higher risk of heart disease and a 25 percent higher risk of stroke than those who do not smoke. For women, the negative effects were even more pronounced.

Now, logically, you might suppose that smoking just one cigarette would carry one-twentieth the risk of smoking a pack, which contains twenty cigarettes. Nope. The researchers found that men who smoked one cigarette per day had nearly half the risk of developing coronary heart disease incurred by those who smoked twenty cigarettes a day; for women who smoked one cigarette daily, the figure was 31 percent of the risk of smokers of twenty per day. These patterns were roughly the same for stroke risk for men and women who smoked just one cigarette daily.

This particular study was a meta-study, a review of other published research whose data was then compiled and critically analyzed. It involved fifty-five publications, encompassing 141 studies, with the goal of determining the relative risk of cigarette smoking for cardiovascular disease.

CARDIOVASCULAR RISKS OF SMOKING

The general mechanisms by which smoking results in cardiovascular events include narrowing of the coronary arteries and an overproduction of blood cells, which together create risk of acute thrombosis (blood clotting). The rapid decline in this risk after a patient stops smoking supports the role of cigarette smoking in blood clotting.

Chemicals in cigarette smoke cause the cells that line the blood vessels to become swollen and inflamed. This can narrow the blood vessels and lead to many cardiovascular conditions. Arteries narrow as plaque builds up, and blood can no longer flow properly to various parts of the heart. Smoking increases the formation of plaque in the coronary arteries.

Peripheral arterial disease (PAD) occurs when blood vessels become narrower and the flow of blood to arms, legs, hands, and feet is reduced. Cells and tissues are deprived of needed oxygen when blood flow is reduced. In extreme cases, an infected limb must be removed. Cigarette smoking is the most common preventable cause of PAD.

Abdominal aortic aneurysm is a bulge or weakened area in the portion of the aorta that is in the abdomen. The aorta is the main artery that carries oxygen-rich blood throughout the body. Smoking is a known cause of early damage to the abdominal aorta, which can lead to an aneurysm. A ruptured abdominal aortic aneurysm is life threatening; almost all deaths from abdominal aortic aneurysms are caused by smoking. Women smokers have a higher risk of dying from an aortic aneurysm than men who smoke. Autopsies have shown early narrowing of the abdominal aorta in young adults who smoked as adolescents.

Atherosclerosis, in which arteries narrow and become less flexible, occurs when fat, cholesterol, and other substances in the blood form plaque that builds up in the walls of arteries. The plaque buildup narrows vessels, so less blood can flow through. When a clot forms in one of these narrow places in an artery around the heart, the heart muscle becomes starved for oxygen. This can cause a heart attack.

Cigarette smoking produces a chronic inflammatory state that contributes to the promotion of fatty plaques in the coronary arteries and elevates levels of biomarkers of inflammation, known powerful predictors of cardiovascular events.

To summarize, smoking damages the heart and blood vessels very quickly, but here's the good news: the damage is repaired quickly as well for most smokers who stop smoking. Even longtime smokers can see rapid health improvements when they quit. Within a year, heart attack risk drops dramatically. Within five years, most smokers cut their risk of stroke to nearly that of a nonsmoker. But again, having even a few cigarettes now and then damages the heart, so the most effective treatment is complete abstinence from cigarette smoking.

A NEW CHAPTER IN AN OLD PROBLEM

Tobacco for smoking was originally cultivated in North America, first by Native American tribes in the mid-Atlantic region and later by British colonists. With that kind of history, you might think there could be nothing new under the sun that could hook a whole new generation of Americans on smoking. Enter vaping, a particularly dangerous trend among young people with real cardiovascular risks. Preliminary research, while not yet definitive, does support the notion there is significant cardiovascular risk to vaping.

Vaping uses so-called e-cigarettes, or battery-operated devices that carry aerosolized vapor that users inhale and then exhale. In that way, they're just like old-school tobacco cigarettes—except there's no tobacco, just a vaporized form of nicotine. Because vaping is so new, having only become popularized in the last decade, there hasn't been enough time to research the cardiovascular effects of it.

Smoking tobacco cigarettes was once promoted as a means of lowering blood pressure and stress. Vaping was originally positioned as an aid for smokers to kick the tobacco habit. It was a risk-benefit roll of the dice with the hope that there wouldn't be any dangerous unintended consequences. As I write this chapter, news has broken of a fifth death due to a mysterious respiratory illness attributed to vaping. This follows the hospitalization of two hundred mostly young people, all experiencing a heretofore unidentified pulmonary affliction.

One theory is that the illness stems from a natural inflammatory response in the lungs, which are filled with blood vessels, due to the introduction of this aerosolized substance. When the lungs encounter bacteria or viruses, this inflammatory response is beneficial, with the body mounting an attack against the foreign and toxic invader. In this case, the body's natural inflammatory response, triggered by the inhaled vapor, becomes the danger. The vaping industry is largely unregulated, and investigators are exploring whether a toxic contaminant might have been inadvertently introduced during the manufacturing process. There's also the still-unanswered question as to what effect breathing in secondhand vaping smoke might have.

This brings us back full circle to the dangers of secondhand smoke. If you live with a smoker (most workers no longer have to worry about fellow employees' smoking), let him or her know that your cardiac health is being putting at risk with every cigarette lit in your presence. Research now shows that exposure to secondhand smoke causes heart disease in nonsmokers. More than thirty-three thousand nonsmokers die every year in the United States from coronary heart disease caused by exposure to secondhand smoke, which leads to heart attacks and strokes in nonsmokers. That works out to about one American dying every fifteen minutes from coronary heart disease, including silent heart disease, caused by somebody else's cigarette smoking habit.

ALCOHOL AND CARDIAC HEALTH

Alcohol—spirits, wine, beer—is so embedded in our culture that it's hard to imagine life without it (although large parts of the world largely refrain from it). In our country, there are religious groups, including the Seventh Day Adventists and Mormons, who reject even the recreational use of any alcohol. Still, alcohol seems to be everywhere in our popular culture, and unlike cigarette smoking, alcohol consumption has not experienced any significant decline over the past sixty years. On the contrary, per capita alcohol consumption in the United States has increased in the past couple of decades to reach a new record of 2.34 gallons of ethanol per capita in 2017.

By any measure the danger of excessive alcohol consumption dwarfs that of all drugs—legal and illegal—combined. In 2018, eighty-eight thousand Americans died because of alcohol abuse, from short-term issues like serious accidents and from long-term health complications, including liver failure, cancer, and heart disease. Of the 21 million people with a substance abuse disorder in 2015, nearly 16 million were in need of treatment for an alcohol problem compared to less than 8 million needing treatment for an illicit drug problem.

A study published in January 2020 in the journal *Alcoholism: Clinical & Experimental Research* found that alcohol-fueled deaths in the United States have doubled over the past twenty years, costing nearly one million lives. All demographic groups (by gender, race, and age) demonstrated increases in deaths by alcohol abuse, but white women registered the largest increases. Why women? The authors speculate that "because women reach higher blood alcohol levels than men of comparable weights after consuming the same amount of alcohol, their body tissues are exposed to more alcohol and acetaldehyde, a toxic metabolite of alcohol, after each drink." This increased sensitivity also makes women more vulnerable to alcohol-related cardiovascular diseases.

The *Journal of the American College of Cardiology* recently reported that ending alcohol abuse would prevent seventy-three thousand clinical episodes of arterial fibrillation, leading to thirty-four thousand fewer heart attacks, and reduce the number of patients with chronic congestive heart failure by ninety-one thousand.

Abusing alcohol, or drinking more than just moderately, doubles the risk of heart attack through several factors. Alcohol contributes to high blood pressure, doubles the risk of atrial fibrillation (irregular, rapid heartbeat), and brings a 2.3-fold increased risk of congestive heart failure—all increasing the risk of heart attack later in life. To frame it another way, the excessive consumption of beer, wine, and spirits directly contributes to a 1.4-fold increase in cardiac episodes. Heavy drinking is also linked to an elevated risk of hypertension, diabetes, cardiovascular disease, stroke, and death after a heart attack, according to the latest research.

However, key to understanding these statistics are the terms "heavy drinking" and "abusive drinking." Unlike cigarette smoking, where the tiniest amount—for example, one cigarette per day (and who smokes only one cigarette every twenty-four hours?)—is dangerous, the consumption of alcohol is much more nuanced. Indeed, as counterintuitive as it might sound, light to moderate drinking can even benefit heart health, as I explain below.

DEFINING TERMS

First, however, let's define terms. According to the Centers for Disease Control and Prevention, a standard drink is equal to 14.0 grams (0.6 ounces) of pure alcohol. Generally, this amount of pure alcohol is found in

- 12 ounces of beer (5 percent alcohol content)
- 8 ounces of malt liquor (7 percent alcohol content)
- 5 ounces of wine (12 percent alcohol content)
- 1.5 ounces, or a "shot," of eighty-proof (40 percent alcohol content) distilled spirits or liquor (for example, gin, rum, vodka, whiskey)

"Moderate" alcohol consumption is defined as up to one drink per day for women and up to two drinks per day for men. This definition refers to the amount consumed on any single day and is not intended as an average over several days. However, the dietary guidelines do not recommend that people who do not drink alcohol start drinking for any reason.

For men, "heavy" drinking is typically defined as consuming fifteen drinks or more per week (using the formula above). For women, heavy drinking is typically defined as consuming eight drinks or more per week. The term "heavy drinking" is defined in terms of a week's consumption versus a day's because, in theory, one could binge drink one day, return to light or moderate drinking for the next six days, and still qualify as a moderate drinker. We'll get more into the difference between heavy drinking and binge drinking in a minute. Suffice it to say, both are significant risk factors for coronary heart disease, but one is much worse.

"Severe alcohol use disorder," also known as alcohol dependence or alcoholism, is a chronic disease, just like drug addiction, with both a genetic and an environmental component. Some of the signs and symptoms of severe alcohol use disorder could include the following:

- Inability to limit drinking
- Continuing to drink despite personal or professional problems
- Needing to drink more to get the same effect
- Wanting a drink so badly you can't think of anything else

CARDIOVASCULAR RISKS AND ALCOHOL

Heavy or extreme alcohol consumption is associated with a vast array of cardiovascular conditions and events, including the following:

- Arrhythmia (irregular heartbeat)
- Cardiomyopathy (a disease of the heart muscle that makes it harder for your heart to efficiently pump blood to the rest of your body)
- Hypertension
- Increased triglyceride levels (associated with clogged arteries)
- Peripheral artery disease
- Death associated with acute cardiovascular events, including sudden cardiac arrest

A concern in the management of any chronic disease, including cardiovascular disease, is drug combining, which increases the risks of adverse effects due to drug interactions. This may include the combination of alcohol with illicit drugs or with prescription drugs. The legal substances may include medications indicated for cardiovascular disorders, which often interact with alcohol to produce negative effects.

A review of data from the American National Health and Nutrition Examination Survey found that the rate of alcohol/prescription drug combination was 41.5 percent. This rate, when adjusted for age (sixty-five years or more), was 77.8 percent. In many cases, the medications in question were for cardiovascular conditions. Another major study on aging found that 72 percent of its approximately thirty-eight hundred participants used medications that interact with alcohol, most often drugs for cardiovascular or neurological conditions. Approximately one in five of these people combined heavy alcohol consumption with anticlotting agents and other drugs for cardiovascular disease. Older people (who are at a higher risk of cardiovascular disease) often have an increased probability of drug/alcohol interaction due to age-related decreases in the ability to absorb and metabolize these compounds.

The effects resulting from cardiovascular drug interactions may include the following:

- Increased blood alcohol levels
- Liver damage
- Gastrointestinal damage and bleeding
- Increased risk of the adverse effects of cardiovascular drugs
- Reduced efficacy of the drugs in question

BINGE DRINKING

In 2018, about 67 million Americans twelve years or older were binge drinkers in the past month, and 16.6 million were heavy drinkers in the past month. What's the difference?

Binge drinking is the quick, high-volume intake of alcohol. The National Institute on Alcohol Abuse and Alcoholism defines binge drinking as consuming five or more drinks for men or four or more drinks for women in about two hours. One research study found that binge drinking six or more cocktails in one evening—servings of hard liquor due to generous pours in bars—increased the risk of heart attack and stroke about 30 percent for the next twenty-four hours and continued a significant increase in the risk of a heart attack or stroke for seven days after the event.

In another study researchers at Harvard University looked at interview data from nearly four thousand people across the United States hospitalized for heart attacks over a three-year period. They looked at the number of alcoholic drinks participants drank in the hour before their heart attack symptoms appeared as well as how much alcohol they drank in the past year. Their findings revealed that people who binge drink are 72 percent more likely to have a heart attack than those who don't.

Now, as alarming as binge drinking sounds, and it is, heavy drinking poses an even greater risk for developing symptoms of heart disease. The daily consumption of large amounts of alcohol, day in and day out, is even worse than the occasional "lost weekend."

BENEFITS OF MODERATE DRINKING

If you have a friend or family member in Alcoholics Anonymous (AA) or who follows another kind of program that requires total abstinence from alcohol of any kind, and you're thinking of lending him or her this book, best to delete this next section. (A few snips of scissors should do the trick.) What I'm about to suggest here—that moderate alcohol consumption actually has a cardiac health benefit—will be viewed by AA and its disciples as nothing less than heresy. I get it, but the science about the benefits of moderate drinking does not lie. Read on, if you dare.

The incidence of heart disease in those who drink moderate amounts of alcohol (no more than two drinks per day for men or one drink per day for women) is lower than in nondrinkers. Over the past several decades, many studies have been published in science journals about how light to moderate drinking of alcohol may be associated with reduced mortality due to heart disease in some populations.

Some researchers have suggested that red wine, consumed moderately, might be especially beneficial. Their thinking is that red wine contains flavonoids and other antioxidants associated with reduced risk of heart disease. Other studies point to moderate consumption of red wine as promoting an increase in HDL ("good") cholesterol, important because of its anticlotting properties.

How alcohol or wine affects cardiovascular risk needs further research, but right now you can rest assured that if you drink moderately, it will not contribute to heart disease and may even benefit your heart health. That's not to suggest that those who do not drink alcohol—because of cultural or religious convictions or because they simply do not like the taste of it or how it makes them feel—should begin consuming alcohol to prevent heart disease. There are other means, including regular

physical activity and eating a whole-foods diet, to achieve the same results. And speaking of diet, alcohol of any kind is loaded with calories.
(There's no such thing as a "beer weight-loss plan" for good reason.)
For all people, alcohol can lower blood sugar, and so for people with
diabetes, it is recommended that any alcohol be consumed with a meal.

AN EXCEPTION TO THE RULE

Earlier we discussed the fundamental difference between cigarette smoking and alcohol consumption. Smoking presents an absolute danger—
even one cigarette a day can pose a risk to cardiac health. On the other
hand, while heavy and binge drinking are absolutely a cardiac risk factor,
light to moderate drinking has proven to be beneficial to the heart.

However, there's one exception to this more nuanced view of
alcohol, and it's for a group of people that crosses all ethnic, racial, and
geographic boundaries—pregnant women. There are no exceptions
and no excuses for pregnant women to drink alcohol, because doing so
can seriously harm the fetus. Fetal alcohol syndrome is a serious birth
defect caused by the consumption of alcohol by the pregnant mother.
About half of babies who suffer from fetal alcohol syndrome have a
heart problem.

LEGAL AND ILLEGAL DRUGS

I recall reading a news story about a gentleman who was so disenchanted
by the results of a recent election that he became a virtual hermit in
our Information Age, refusing to read, hear, or see any news accounts
about anything. He's probably the only person at this point who hasn't
heard that the nation continues to be gripped by a drug problem of epic
proportions.

For the record, let's recap what this unprecedented drug epidemic
looks like. From 1999 through 2016, the age-adjusted rate of drug-
overdose deaths in the United States more than tripled from 6.1 per
100,000 to 19.8 per 100,000. The only comparable recent epidemic
in modern times to spike so dramatically with such devastating conse-

quences was HIV/AIDS, and, as noted earlier, opioids have killed many more than AIDS.

As with the obesity epidemic, the opioid epidemic is a worldwide problem but is much worse in the United States than in any other country. When it comes to overprescribing prescription painkillers, the United States leads the way. A recent study on overprescription of opioids by U.S. physicians showed that Americans are seven times more likely to get opioids after surgery than Swedish patients, and not only more pills but higher dosages as well.

CARDIAC PROBLEMS WITH OPIOID USE

Opioids mimic the body's natural endorphins by binding to pain receptors to inhibit their signaling to the brain. Some of the earliest drugs, including heroin, are opioids. These drugs have neurological effects besides analgesia, which may include euphoria, lethargy, respiratory problems, and withdrawal symptoms. However, in excessive doses, opioids' action on the nervous system can produce several other effects, including sedation, depressed breathing, seizures, confusion, vomiting, pinpoint pupils, and stupor. Death from an opioid overdose most often occurs during an opioid-induced stupor, in which the respiratory drive becomes so thoroughly depressed that breathing simply slows down or even stops.

Given the national spotlight on deaths due to opioid overdose, the many cardiac problems caused by these substances have received little attention. However, opioids are now associated with several kinds of potentially life-threatening heart problems.

Opioid use over time can increase the risk of cardiovascular disease by increasing the concentrations of low-density lipoproteins and free triglycerides in the body, both associated with increased risks of atherosclerosis, stroke, and heart attack. A study comparing 117 coronary artery bypass patients who also abused opioids with 208 similar patients who did not abuse these substances found that low-density lipoprotein and average triglyceride levels were significantly higher in the substance-abusing patients.

While opioids by themselves have little effect on the ability of the heart muscle to contract forcefully, this ability can be suppressed when opioids are combined with benzodiazepines (drugs like Valium). This combination is not uncommon in people chronically taking opioids. In people who have an underlying heart problem that produces some degree of weakness in cardiac function, such as cardiomyopathy, the combination of an opioid and a benzodiazepine can precipitate overt heart failure.

Bradycardia, or a slow heart rate, is seen fairly frequently in people taking opioids. Generally, this condition is due to a slowing of impulses from the sinus node, as is seen in sick sinus syndrome. Opioid bradycardia rarely causes symptoms at rest, but it can lead to poor exercise tolerance, since the heart rate may be incapable of increasing normally with exercise.

Opioid use is a risk factor in vasodilation, or dilation of the blood vessels. This condition can cause hypotension (low blood pressure). Because opioids also can produce bradycardia along with vasodilation, a person on opioids who stands up quickly may experience a sudden drop in blood pressure—a condition called orthostatic hypotension.

Two opioids in particular (methadone and buprenorphine) can induce a phenomenon on the electrocardiogram (EKG) called QT prolongation. In some people, QT prolongation can be associated with a dangerous form of ventricular tachycardia called torsades de pointes. This type of cardiac arrhythmia commonly produces episodes of severe lightheadedness, temporary loss of consciousness, or even sudden death.

Atrial fibrillation is a rapid, irregular heart rhythm caused by a disrupted electrical signal in the heart's atria (the upper cardiac chambers). People who take opioids are at a higher risk of the condition. People with atrial fibrillation have a relatively high incidence of stroke and possibly of heart attacks.

Infectious endocarditis is an infection of the heart valves, a relatively rare but life-threatening condition seen mainly in the elderly. Recently, however, many more young people than ever before—particularly young, white women—have been diagnosed with the condition. The common denominator among these young people with endocarditis? They have abused intravenous opioids, especially heroin. Infectious endocarditis has a high mortality rate, and survivors are commonly left with chronic cardiac disease.

THE PERFECT HEART ATTACK DRUG

Here's some good news about the opioid epidemic: the number of opioid prescriptions actually peaked in 2012 and has declined ever since. Opioids, both legal (notably, oxycodone) and illicit (notably, heroin), initially fueled the nation's twenty-first-century drug epidemic. Cocaine, on its own or mixed with illicit synthetic forms of the powerful opioid fentanyl, has overtaken opioids, killing nearly thirty-two thousand Americans in 2018.

As cocaine use increases in the United States, researchers have begun to examine associated demographic trends. Using nationally representative survey data encompassing responses about substance use collected from 281,242 people between 2011 and 2015, they found that cocaine use had increased the most among three groups: women, people between the ages of eighteen and twenty-five, and people over age fifty.

An Australian study presented at the American Heart Association's Scientific Sessions in 2012 was the first to document cardiovascular abnormalities in seemingly healthy regular cocaine users long after the immediate effects of cocaine had worn off. Researchers—who called cocaine "the perfect heart attack drug"—showed how users had higher rates of multiple factors associated with higher risks of heart attack and stroke:

- 30 to 35 percent increase in aortic stiffening,
- 8 mmHg higher systolic blood pressure, and
- 18 percent greater thickness of the heart's left ventricle wall.

The abuse of cocaine is also linked to the increased risk of infections of heart muscle and other cardiac tissues. This leads to conditions such as endocarditis, which in turn may result in increased risk of hospital readmission for conditions such as stroke, arrythmia, heart attack, and heart failure.

Cocaine is the illegal drug most often associated with visits to U.S. hospital emergency departments. Cocaine use has been associated with chest pain and myocardial infarction. In 2011, it was involved in an estimated 40.3 percent of illicit-drug-related emergency department visits (505,224 visits) versus about 36.4 percent (455,668 visits) for marijuana and about 20.6 percent (258,482 visits) for heroin.

Cocaine-induced heart attacks are not just a risk for individuals who've used the drug for years. A first-time user can experience a cocaine-induced heart attack. Cocaine use quadruples sudden death in users fifteen to forty-nine years of age, due primarily to resulting cardiovascular disease.

The most significant damage to the heart, however, may be occurring silently. This lasting damage may be difficult to detect. A 2011 study found that medical tests rarely show damage to a cocaine user's blood vessels or heart.

The use of cocaine also complicates cardiovascular treatments. For example, people who use cocaine cannot take beta-blockers, a critical medication for lowering blood pressure by blocking the effects of the hormone adrenaline. Blocking adrenaline slows the heart rate and allows the heart to pump less forcefully. In individuals who've used cocaine, beta-blockers may actually lead to greater blood vessel constriction, which can increase blood pressure even more.

COCAINE-FENTANYL COCKTAIL

In 2016, the number of overdose deaths involving cocaine almost doubled from two years prior, jumping from 5,892 to 11,316. Forty percent of these deaths also involved a newly emerging synthetic version of fentanyl, an opioid fifty times more potent than morphine. This latest wave of substance abuse is too new for much research to have been done on its effect on cardiac health beyond, of course, those cases resulting in death by overdose. But the most recent statistics show clearly that cocaine and fentanyl are being mixed together in a deadly cocktail, often without the knowledge of buyers, who think they are getting pure cocaine.

Fentanyl first captured the nation's attention when the death of pop music star Prince in 2016 was determined to have been caused by an overdose of the drug. However, the overdose was from a prescribed form of the drug, which he was taking for pain from numerous injuries suffered while performing. The cheap, synthetic forms of the drug flooding into the United States are imported mainly from legal and illicit sources in China.

How the nation will emerge from the triple wave of the drug crisis of the last decade—prescription pain killers, cocaine, and fentanyl—is anyone's guess at this point. In the case of the latter, pushers haven't even had time to come up with a street idiom for the drug—they call it fentanyl too.

Research into marijuana and its potential to affect cardiac health is also lacking. Banned as a Schedule 1 drug (right up there with heroin, LSD, and methamphetamine), which hampered its study by medical researchers, marijuana, or cannabis, as a risk factor in cardiovascular disease is just coming under the microscope as individual states have begun to decriminalize its recreational use.

14

ANXIETY, STRESS, AND SLEEP IMPAIRMENT

Earlier in the book, I introduced three of my cardiology patients: Nathan, age thirty-six, the video game developer with a poor diet and sedentary lifestyle; Angela, age fifty-seven, the cerebral rocket scientist with type 2 diabetes; and Frank, forty-five, the apparel entrepreneur with a Type A personality and hypertension. Each of them had a different primary risk factor for silent heart disease (and coronary heart disease). However, they also shared another common risk factor: they all suffered from anxiety, stress, and sleep impairment.

There's nothing coincidental in all three of these patients having these common risk factors, because I believe the vast majority of people who suffer from coronary heart disease also suffer to some degree from one or more of these conditions. I literally have seen tens of thousands of patients over the course of my sixty years in practice as a cardiologist, and there's no doubt in my mind that anxiety-related conditions are among the most common risk factors in these patients.

Until recently, the medical community didn't believe that these conditions contributed directly to the risk of heart disease. After all, stress to some degree is part of everyday life. Running late for the important client meeting, an unexpected car-repair bill, a family member with a substance abuse disorder—all are examples of common, everyday stressors. Likewise, the idea that an impaired sleep condition like insomnia might be a primary factor in coronary heart disease was viewed skeptically by physicians and the public alike. As long as you got yourself to work every day, you could always compensate for your restless nights during the workweek by catching up with extra sleep during the weekend—or so the thinking at the time went.

Today, there is substantial evidence that stress, anxiety, and sleep impairment are conditions that not only commonly occur in patients with coronary heart disease (CHD) but may actually have a causal effect as important as cigarette smoking, high blood pressure, and high cholesterol, the three "classic" risk factors for heart disease. What's more, stress, anxiety, and sleep impairment can also trigger development of other risk factors, such as obesity and substance abuse.

Stress, anxiety, and sleep impairment often have similar causes, so it is important to understand all of them because the most effective treatment depends on an accurate diagnosis. In this final chapter of Part II, we'll address the ones that are most relevant as risk factors for silent heart disease.

STRESS VERSUS ANXIETY

The terms "stress" and "anxiety" are often used interchangeably by the public. Phrasing such as "I'm really anxious to hear back about my job interview" or "the long commute is stressing me out" are common colloquialisms. However, it must be recognized that stress and anxiety are two separate conditions, although they overlap in significant ways.

The best way of thinking about the difference is that stress is caused by external factors (lack of money, overbearing boss, crowded freeway), while anxiety is usually caused by internal factors—your view of or fears about the world around you. Both conditions can be treated, often with the same or similar treatment protocols, including medications, exercise, meditation, and psychological counseling. But for treatment to be most effective, it's necessary to understand the differences between these conditions as well.

Stress is basically the quite normal response our bodies have to any change in our environment. Such changes can be either positive or negative and lie along a continuum in terms of being within or outside our control. The less control we have over the situation that is creating the stress we are experiencing, the more intense our stress reaction is likely to be. Not only do we experience stress as a response to even positive changes in our lives, but the stress reaction itself is also a positive and beneficial response at times.

The human body is designed to react to stress effectively. You probably have heard of the "fight-or-flight response," which generates physiological changes in order for the body to successfully react to stressful situations. When this natural, healthy stress response is activated over a prolonged period, however, it can cause physical and emotional wear and tear on our bodies. Such a negative state of stress, or distress, can lead to serious health problems if left untreated. Many times, it is the physical symptoms of stress that drive people to the doctor. Work, the demands of family, social relationships, and financial problems are some of the leading causes of stress.

The following is a list of common responses to untreated stress:

- High blood pressure
- Digestive issues
- Headaches
- Muscle aches and pains
- Tremors
- Sleep disturbances
- Depressed immune system (frequent colds, viruses)
- Skin problems (rashes, hives)
- Memory problems (forgetfulness)
- Lack of focus and concentration
- Bouts of depression

Similarly, do you do any of the following when you're "stressed out"?

- Eat to calm down
- Speak and eat very fast
- Drink alcohol or smoke
- Rush around but not get much done
- Work too much
- Procrastinate
- Sleep too little, too much, or both
- Slow down
- Try to do too many things at once

Ultimately, people feel and react to stress in different ways. Your stress reaction depends on specific environmental factors in your life, although certainly society as a whole can be under stress. For example, much has been written about how the benignly termed Information Age—gee, who doesn't like information?—has created a modern-day milieu where we're never really disconnected from the Internet of Things. Just the other day I marveled at how a young man, who appeared to be a professional dog walker because of the half dozen canines he was walking, could not bring himself to stop texting on his smartphone—never mind that in doing so he posed a danger to his charges, himself, other pedestrians, and the vehicular traffic all around him. This inability to unplug from the Internet can easily cross the line into obsessive-compulsive behavior.

How much stress you experience and how you react to it can lead to a wide variety of health problems—and that's why it's critical to know what you can do about it. Excessive stress can contribute to everything from high blood pressure to asthma, ulcers, irritable bowel syndrome, and coronary heart disease.

ANXIETY DISORDERS

If you feel anxious now and then, that's perfectly normal. Like stress, a little anxiety can spur you to take positive action that may benefit your health, such as getting screening tests, doing regular exercise, or embracing a healthy diet. But excessive worrying can have the opposite effect.

Anxiety is more than just feeling stressed or worried. Anxious feelings are a normal reaction to feeling under pressure, and usually these symptoms disappear once the stressful situation has passed, or the "stressor" is removed. However, for some people these anxious feelings happen for no apparent reason or continue even after the stressful event has passed. For a person experiencing clinical anxiety, anxious feelings often cannot be brought under control easily.

Anxiety can be a serious condition that makes it hard for a person to cope with daily life. There are many types of anxiety, and many people with anxiety experience symptoms of more than one type. In fact, living with coronary heart disease is one of many stressors that may trigger anxiety. Anxiety is common, and the sooner people get help, the sooner they can recover.

The symptoms of anxiety can often develop gradually over time. Given that we all experience some anxious feelings, it can be hard to know how much is too much. In order to be diagnosed with an anxiety condition, a person's anxiety must have a disabling impact on his or her life.

Anxiety can be expressed in different ways, such as uncontrollable worry, intense fear (phobias or panic attacks), upsetting dreams, or flashbacks to a traumatic event. Some common symptoms of anxiety include the following:

- Hot and cold flashes
- Racing heart
- Tightening of the chest
- Snowballing worries
- Shortness of breath or difficulty breathing
- Obsessive thinking and compulsive behavior
- Feeling restless, wound up, or on edge
- Being easily fatigued
- Difficulty concentrating; mind going blank
- Irritability
- Difficulty controlling feelings of worry
- Sleep problems, such as insomnia or interrupted sleep

So, how can you tell if you're just going through an especially stressful episode in your life or you have a clinical form of anxiety? One common form, generalized anxiety disorder, is characterized by at least six months of excessive worrying or feeling anxious about several unrelated events or activities almost every day. About 5 percent of adults in the general population meet the criteria for generalized anxiety disorder, but the incidence is higher among people diagnosed with coronary artery disease (11 percent) or heart failure (13 percent).

PANIC ATTACKS

In a panic attack, an intense rush of fear or anxiety can make one feel just like he or she is having a heart attack, with chest pain, shortness of breath, sweating, nausea, lightheadedness, and a racing or pounding heart. These frightening episodes propel many people to seek emergency care, where oftentimes careful testing uncovers no evidence of a heart problem. Instead, these people receive a diagnosis of what's known as noncardiac chest pain (NCCP), which is surprisingly common.

As many as one in three people experience NCCP at some point in their lives, according to a 2017 review article in the journal *Psychosomatics*. While some cases end up being traced to a gastrointestinal or muscle-related problem, people with NCCP often have very high levels of anxiety, says Harvard psychiatrist Dr. Christopher Celano. "If you're having chest pain, you should definitely go to the emergency room to make sure you're not having a heart attack," he says.

But if it's not a heart attack, what's next? It's not uncommon for people with an anxiety disorder—especially those who have panic attacks—to continue having symptoms and to end up back in the emergency room. Cardiologists see this problem all the time. The best way to tell the difference between a heart attack and a panic attack is through diagnostic testing.

IMPACT ON CARDIAC HEALTH

Ironically, those who think they are suffering from a heart attack, even though it is in fact a panic attack, may actually be contributing unknowingly to silent heart disease. That is, researchers have reported that heart patients who have generalized anxiety disorder—constant, pervasive worrying, even about mundane matters—are more likely to have heart attacks and serious heart problems than patients who don't have these symptoms. In a recent study, Canadian researchers analyzed studies of people treated in emergency departments for chest pain. Their conclusion: about one in five of those who underwent cardiovascular testing had experienced a panic attack, not a heart attack.

It's not totally clear yet why heart disease and anxiety are connected, but acute anxiety may actually be associated with acute heart attacks. Generalized anxiety disorder is associated with surges of the stress hormone cortisol and an outpouring of other chemicals involved in the fight-or-flight response. That in turn appears to make heart attacks and other cardiac events more likely. But why?

Let's dig a little deeper into the relationship between cardiac health and cortisol. A review published in June 2017 in the journal *Frontiers in Human Neuroscience* concluded that inflammation is a common pathway of stress-related diseases. In a fight-or-flight emergency situation, the stress hormone cortisol affects nonessential functions, like your immune response and digestion. The hormone also fuels the production of glucose, or blood sugar, boosting energy to the large muscles, while inhibiting insulin production and narrowing arteries, which forces the heart to pump harder to start the stressor response.

Another hormone, adrenaline, is also released in these situations, which tells the body to increase heart and respiratory rates and to expand airways to push more oxygen into muscles. Your body also makes glycogen, or stored glucose (sugar), available to power muscles. In addition, stress decreases lymphocytes, white blood cells that are part of the inflammatory immune systems.

Pro-inflammatory cytokines usually do their job and then disappear, but when stress is chronic, they are "upregulated" in your system—meaning the cycle of stress and inflammatory response gets habituated in the body. Over time, these cytokines may perpetuate themselves. That's when inflammation starts to have deleterious effects on the body. And while no one is completely sure why that happens (there are many mechanisms responsible for diseases), many conditions have chronic, low-level inflammation in common.

A hyped-up sympathetic nervous system—the response that primes your body to fight or flee—also works to constrict blood vessels, which forces your heart to work harder and raises blood pressure.

Inflammation is at the core of the development of atherosclerosis, a precursor to heart disease. Ironically, in its initial response to danger, cortisol is a potent anti-inflammatory that functions to mobilize glucose reserves for energy and modulate inflammation. On a psychological level, cortisol also may facilitate the consolidation of fear-based memories for future survival and avoidance of danger. Ultimately, however, a prolonged or exaggerated stress response may perpetuate cortisol dysfunction, widespread inflammation, and pain.

Another theory as to the correlation and possible causal effect between anxiety and coronary heart disease is that people with generalized anxiety disorder tend to have low levels of omega-3 fatty acids, which have some properties that may fend off heart disease. Another theory is that the real culprit is depression, despite the best efforts by researchers to tease apart depression and anxiety and investigate them separately. The boundary between major depression and generalized anxiety disorder is inherently fuzzy, at both the biological and psychological levels.

Still another possibility is that anxious patients with coronary heart disease may be less likely to seek preventive medical care, possibly due to an avoidant coping strategy. It is also possible that there exists a common background origin to stress and anxiety symptoms and the risk of cardiovascular disease—some still to-be-discovered interplay of genetic factors.

So, while scientists have not been able to pinpoint the exact reason for the correlation, there's little doubt that high stress and anxiety can set the stage for heart disease. To frame it another way, those of us who perceive a lot of stress in our lives are at higher risk for heart attack and other cardiovascular problems over the long term.

Several studies have shown that about a quarter of people with cardiovascular disease have some kind of anxiety problem, and in some cases the anxiety seems to make the heart condition worse. The latest evidence comes from a new study of siblings in Sweden, published in 2019 in the *British Medical Journal*. Researchers identified about 137,000 people who had been diagnosed with stress-related disorders. Then the researchers identified about 171,000 of their brothers and sisters with similar upbringings and genes but no anxiety disorder. Next they compared the siblings' rates of cardiovascular disease, including heart attacks, cardiac arrest, and blood clots, over a number of years. The Swedes who had a stress disorder, it turns out, had significantly higher rates of heart problems compared to their siblings. "We saw [about] a 60 percent increased risk of having any cardiovascular events" within the first year after being diagnosed, says Unnur A. Valdimarsdóttir, a researcher with the Karolinska Institute and professor of epidemiology at the University of Iceland. Over the longer term, the increased risk was about 30 percent.

So, if stress and anxiety are normal parts of life, when do they become a risk factor for silent heart disease and coronary events? The problem is not that we occasionally experience the fight-or-flight stress response, an essential mechanism humans have evolved as the dominant animal species. When in danger, our ancestors counted on their bodies to smartly increase their heart rate and blood pressure to take immediate action—such as fleeing from a hungry predator with very large teeth. The problem comes if you start to experience these stress response "activations" even when there's not an imminent threat—the lion is nowhere to be seen.

IMPAIRED SLEEP

Of all the reasons to get a good night's sleep, protecting your heart might not be top of mind. But maybe it should be. Sleep duration has decreased 1.5 to 2 hours per night per person in the last fifty years. But several recent studies show links between shortened sleep duration, defined as less than six hours of sleep, and increased risk of heart disease.

A 2011 *European Heart Journal* review of fifteen medical studies involving almost 475,000 people found that short sleepers had a 48 percent increased risk of developing or dying from coronary heart disease in a seven to twenty-five-year follow-up period (depending on the study) and a 15 percent greater risk of developing or dying from stroke during this same time. Interestingly, long sleepers—those who averaged nine or more hours a night—also showed a 38 percent increased risk of developing or dying from CHD and a 65 percent increased risk of stroke.

Researchers caution that the mechanisms behind shortened and prolonged sleep and heart disease aren't completely understood. "Lack of sleep doesn't necessarily cause heart disease," says Phyllis Zee, MD, PhD, professor of neurology and director of the Sleep Disorders Program at Northwestern University's Feinberg School of Medicine. "It really increases the risk factors for heart disease."

Part of the reason for the lack of understanding is that sleep's effects on the heart is a relatively new area of study. Another is that measuring sleep is complicated. Many sleep studies rely on self-reporting, which may not always be accurate. Having your sleep measured involves wearing an activity monitor, which quite likely may change your usual sleep pattern.

Good quality sleep decreases the work of your heart, as blood pressure and heart rate go down at night. People who are sleep-deprived show less variability in their heart rate, meaning that instead of fluctuating normally, the heart rate usually stays elevated. "That is not a good sign," Zee says. "That looks like heightened stress."

Zee also identifies a host of other factors. Lack of sleep can increase insulin resistance, a risk factor for the development of type 2 diabetes and heart disease. Shortened sleep can increase C-reactive protein (CRP), which is released with stress and inflammation. "If your CRP is high, it's a risk factor for cardiovascular and heart disease," says Zee. Shortened sleep also interferes with appetite regulation. "So you may end up eating more or eating foods that are less healthy for your heart," Zee says.

Individuals may have biological or psychological traits that increase their likelihood of developing acute sleep problems when faced with precipitating factors, such as stress or anxiety. In an attempt to compensate for poor sleep, individuals may unwittingly engage in behaviors that ultimately perpetuate their sleep problems.

LESS IS MORE

Is there an ideal amount of sleep? The short answer is yes. While each of us is of course unique physiologically to some degree, by and large research has shown that the average person requires eight hours of restful sleep. Any less or any more is considered impaired sleep.

To be clear, spending more time in bed to compensate for poor sleep can have the unintended effect of disrupting sleep/wake cycles, decreasing sleep efficiency, and creating a conditioned association between being in bed and being awake. Others may compensate for poor sleep by taking daytime naps (which decreases the urge to sleep the following night) or increasing caffeine intake. Over time, individuals may come to regard nighttime as a frustrating struggle, which increases physiological activation and further decreases the likelihood of entering a comfortable sleep state.

INSOMNIA AND CORONARY HEART DISEASE

Insomnia, a common type of impaired sleep that's generally thought of as an inability to fall or stay asleep on at least three days in a week, is due to overarousal that persists into the evening and night. This means that the sympathetic nervous system has increased activity with increased release of stress hormones such as cortisol. Chronic activation of the stress system may have effects such as increasing insulin resistance and contributing to psychological problems such as depression and anxiety. Depression itself can increase the risk of cardiovascular disease. Insomnia appears to be associated with impaired glucose metabolism, and this may damage the cardiovascular system and contribute to the development of cardiovascular disease.

Dysregulation of the sympathetic nervous system has been linked to high blood pressure, cardiac arrhythmias, and heart failure. Increased levels of C-reactive protein have been linked to severe insomnia in men. Elevated CRP levels have been implicated in the development of plaques in arteries. Very chronic insomnia has been associated with increased risk of high blood pressure. This is especially the case when patients with insomnia also get less than six hours of sleep per night.

The potential relationship between insomnia and cardiovascular disease may have to do with the insomnia along with the potential effect of short sleep duration. This state of hyperarousal involves increased systemic inflammation and a disruption of stress regulators in the pituitary-adrenal glands. These factors then impact various pathways to cardiovascular disease such as increasing heart rate and blood pressure, increasing the development of plaques in the arteries, and increasing resistance to insulin and raising levels of lipids such as cholesterol in the blood.

SLEEP DURATION VERSUS SLEEP INTERRUPTION

Most studies investigating the correlation between impaired sleep as a risk factor in coronary heart disease have used duration as the only measure of sleep. However, more recent evidence demonstrates that aspects of sleep other than sleep duration are also important to investigate.

A recent report found that the combination of sleep duration and sleep disturbance was a better predictor of coronary heart disease risk than sleep duration alone. The Whitehall II study was a major longitudinal study tracking the health of more than ten thousand workers, ages thirty-five to fifty-five, from twenty departments of the British Civil Service across fifteen years. Although both sleep duration and sleep disturbance were associated with increased coronary heart disease risk, only sleep disturbance remained significant after adjustment for environmental and genetic factors. Upon closer examination, it appeared that there was an interaction between sleep disturbance and sleep duration, such that those with short sleep duration were at increased risk of coronary heart disease only if they also reported subjective sleep disturbance. The Whitehall II data echo findings of earlier studies that reported that individuals with insomnia, one type of sleep disturbance, were at increased risk of hypertension if they also reported short sleep duration. Thus, in this study as well others, an indicator of cardiovascular disease is associated with increased sleep disturbance in the context of short sleep duration.

The most common reason for sleep interruption was urination during the night. Also, for female patients, self-perceived poor health, co-morbidities, and depression were also contributing factors. Insomnia was reported by 32 percent of patients with heart failure in a recent study. The most mentioned problems with sleep were difficulty falling asleep, difficulty staying asleep, and waking up too early.

Factors that studies have found are correlated with insomnia are depression, anxiety, marital status (divorced, widowed), and something known in the medical profession as "dyspnea," sometimes known colloquially as "air hunger." Patients with dyspnea describe it as a shortness of breath or an inability to breathe in enough air.

SLEEP APNEA

Sleep apnea is a prevalent condition characterized by frequent pauses in breathing when a person sleeps. According to the National Sleep Foundation, more than 18 million people in the United States suffer from sleep apnea, many of whom have not been officially diagnosed. When sleep apnea goes unnoticed, people cannot receive the treatment they need. Initially, this can lead to daily issues such as headaches, fatigue, and poor memory. Over time, sleep apnea can lead to more serious health concerns, including diabetes, hypertension, and stroke.

The relationship between sleep apnea and cardiovascular disease most likely stems from repeated episodes of decreased blood oxygen levels, as breathing is cut off by the closing of the upper airway, and the repeated stimulation of the heart as the brain arouses the body to increase the tone of the airway muscles so that breathing can be restored. Over time this takes a toll on the heart and blood vessels. The ways in which insomnia may negatively affect the vascular system are not as well understood but most likely involve processes such as increased sympathetic nervous system activity associated with overarousal and increased inflammation.

Sleep apnea is estimated to affect 14 to 49 percent of the adult population; moderate to severe sleep apnea is present in around 10 percent of adults above thirty years of age, and its prevalence increases sharply with age. Sleep apnea is more common among men than in women.

WHAT CAUSES SLEEP APNEA?

There are a number of factors that increase risk, including having a small upper airway (or large tongue, tonsils, or uvula), being overweight, having a recessed chin, small jaw, or large overbite, having a large neck size (seventeen inches or greater in a man; sixteen inches or greater in a woman), smoking and alcohol use, being age forty or older, and being of certain ethnicities (African American, Pacific Islander, and Hispanic). Also, sleep apnea seems to run in some families, suggesting a possible genetic basis.

How can you tell if you have sleep apnea? Chronic snoring is a strong indicator of the condition and should be evaluated by a health professional. Since people with sleep apnea tend to be sleep deprived, they may suffer from sleepiness and a wide range of other symptoms such as difficulty concentrating, depression, irritability, sexual dysfunction, learning and memory difficulties, and falling asleep while at work, on the phone, or driving. Left untreated, sleep apnea can lead to disturbed sleep, excessive sleepiness during the day, high blood pressure, heart attack, congestive heart failure, cardiac arrhythmia, stroke, or depression.

There's also a disturbing association between sleep apnea and diabetes, which is a leading risk factor in coronary heart disease. When a person is asleep, the parasympathetic nervous system—also called the "rest-and-digest" system—dominates, resulting in a slowdown of heart rate, blood pressure, respiration rate, gut movement, other bodily functions, body temperature, and basal metabolism. However, if sleep is disturbed too often, this rest-and-digest system is never triggered, resulting in a heightened load on the circulatory system, an elevated basal metabolism rate, and a higher level of stress hormones.

Research indicates the association between sleep and diabetes may be described as a vicious circle, where sleep disorders favor the development of type 2 diabetes. On the other hand, diabetes itself, when accompanied by poor metabolic control, is mostly followed by sleep disorders.

TREATMENTS (ONE SIZE DOES NOT FIT ALL)

While the latest scientific research clearly indicates a link between cardiac health and stress, anxiety, and impaired sleep (including insomnia and sleep apnea), the medical profession is still playing catch-up. Because these conditions are so intertwined, their effects are more difficult to measure than the so-called classic coronary heart disease risk factors, such as high blood pressure, high levels of low-density lipoproteins, diabetes, and smoking. There's no litmus test to determine if a patient's stress, anxiety, or impaired sleep has crossed the line between inconvenient and potentially life threatening. And there is no single way to treat these conditions. It's different for everybody.

My patient Nathan, the thirty-six-year-old video game developer, had sleep apnea in addition to poor diet and a sedentary lifestyle. For his sleep apnea, I recommended a physician colleague specializing in bioesthetic dentistry. Once Nathan's mouth cavity was X-rayed, he was diagnosed with temporomandibular disorder, a condition characterized by a misalignment of the upper and lower jaw. Nathan's abnormal jaw position caused a serous breathing problem when he slept. The solution? A customized ultralight orthodontic device that fit behind his teeth, making it nearly invisible, which over the course of a year properly realigned his jaw and cured his sleep apnea.

Angela, the fifty-seven-year-old NASA engineer with type 2 diabetes, had her first panic attack just one week before her team's launch of a Mars landing rover. Needless to say, there was incredible pressure to get everything 110 percent correct, which was all the more intense because it was her first project as team leader. Her treatment was a personalized regimen of relaxation training that included a combination of tai chi, mindfulness meditation, and breathing exercises. We also discovered that her sleep was constantly being interrupted by her need to go to the bathroom. A tried-and-true medication for incontinency quickly solved that problem.

Frank, our gregarious, combative forty-five-year-old entrepreneur, still struggled with high blood pressure even with medications. After questioning at length about his sleeping habits, he admitted that he frequently struggled with insomnia. He solution was to "calm his nerves" with a couple of vodka martinis every night after work, but in fact his constant alcohol intake was only contributing to his insomnia. While the alcohol initially made him doze off in front of the TV, it also dehydrated him, compelling him to wake up frequently to quench his thirst. The solution was to limit his alcohol intake altogether and to drink no alcohol two to three hours before going to bed. With this new regimen, we broke his bad habit of falling asleep in front of the TV and actually got him to start scheduling his sleep time. Now, while the thought of scheduling bedtime might drive some people crazy, it was just what Type A personality Frank needed.

Still, Frank needed more. I had a hunch that he might have a clinical anxiety disorder, possibly borderline depression. Consultation with his wife revealed that he exhibited some classic signs of depression, including bouts of anger and reckless behavior, notably driving dangerously after a few cocktails. (Depression is often overlooked in men as a risk factor for not only coronary heart disease but suicide as well. Men suffering from depression are four times more likely to commit suicide than women.)

In short, Frank needed psychological counseling. I knew he wouldn't have the patience for Freudian-based psychoanalysis, so instead I recommended a colleague who specialized in interpersonal therapy, which helps people find new ways of getting along with others and resolving loss, change, and conflict in relationships.

After a year of controlling his blood pressure, insomnia, and anxiety, Frank made measurable improvement across the board in all of his cardiac biomarkers (more about these biomarkers in Part III). Was he a new man? No, he was still the same Frank that those who knew him well couldn't help but like.

"You know, Harold, I'm thinking of joining an improv comedy troupe on weekends as a relaxation technique. What do you think?" Frank asked during one of his regular six-month checkups. "And by the way, how's the blood pressure?"

"I'm happy to report your blood pressure is normal. No kidding!" I said.

PART II: TAKEAWAYS

In Part II of the book, we learned there are many different kinds of risk factors for silent heart disease and coronary heart disease in general. Medical science has divided the risk factors into two broad categories: genetic, also known as "nature," and environmental, also known as "nurture." Essentially, you're born with the nature risk factors, inherited as they are from your parents. The nurture risk factors are acquired after you're born and are to a large degree the results of your circumstances and behavioral and lifestyle choices.

Let's quickly review each of these risk factors.

NATURE

Genetic

- Family history: When it comes to a genetic predisposition for silent heart disease, your family history is a complex factor in determining your overall risk. However, your first-degree relatives—your parents and siblings—are the most important in determining your own risk factors. If they had heart disease before the age of fifty-five, chances are you will too. If there is an upside to bad genes, it is that the genetic effect tends to become diluted later in life. So while you cannot escape your genes, it is possible to stay ahead of them with appropriate lifestyle changes and treatments.
- Age and gender: Older men have the highest risk of silent heart disease. Men are ten times more likely than women to develop a

heart attack prior to the age of forty-five and seven times more likely to do so between ages fifty-five and sixty-four. However, the playing field levels out with age, with sixty-five- to seventy-four-year-old men only twice as likely as women to be felled by heart disease. Bottom line: Heart disease remains the number one killer of men and women in the United States.

- High LDL cholesterol: There is a significant correlation between the level of LDL cholesterol and the risk of developing coronary heart disease. Since 1984, it has been clear among medical experts that lowering elevated levels of cholesterol in the blood will reduce the risk of heart disease. This fatty, yellowish substance has been identified as the leading cause of arteriosclerotic plaque buildup in the coronary arteries.

- High blood pressure: While the incidence of heart disease has declined over the past half century (despite its remaining the number one killer of adult men and women in the United States), new research shows that heart disease once again is spiking in the United States because of increased rates of high blood pressure. Genetic risk factors, including family history, age, race, and gender, all figure into abnormally high blood pressure. As with cholesterol, high blood pressure can also be caused by environmental factors, including poor diet and lack of exercise.

- Diabetes and kidney disease: Diabetes puts patients at huge risk for heart disease. Heart attacks and other cardiovascular complications cause the deaths of nearly three out of every four people with diabetes, compared with just one in four people in the general population. Kidney disease is also an inherited risk factor, and the two conditions can be interrelated. Heart disease is the most common cause of death among people who have kidney disease. People with diabetes and kidney disease may also be more at risk for silent heart disease and silent heart attacks—the ones that mostly go unnoticed—because both diseases can cause damage to the peripheral nervous system. As a result, researchers believe that persons with diabetes and kidney disease often simply can't feel when they have a heart attack.

NURTURE

Environment and Behavior

- Diet: While heart disease has remained the number one cause of death in America, over the last half century the percentage of U.S. citizens succumbing to the disease has gone down. A large part of the reason is that Americans eat a much more "heart-healthy" diet and are much more conscious of the need to lower their cholesterol levels than was the case just a generation ago. Still, we eat too much saturated fat, sugar, and salt, which all contribute to heart disease. Over the decades, as diet fads have come and gone, one type of diet has stood the test of time: the Mediterranean diet, characterized by the consumption of lots of fresh fruits and vegetables, the avoidance of red meat, and an emphasis on fresh seafood and olive oil as the primary sources of fat.
- Sedentary lifestyle: Research gathered on the benefits of exercise since the fitness craze took off in the 1970s clearly shows that keeping the body in motion by exercising regularly can help to lower cholesterol, still the primary cause of silent heart disease. It's more beneficial to move throughout the day—every hour or so—than it is to exercise strenuously at the beginning or end of each day or just on weekends. Men over fifty years old (the group most at risk for silent heart disease) who engage in vigorous leisure-time exercise—even just a brisk walk thirty minutes a day—reportedly have 50 percent fewer heart attacks than their sedentary peers. Exercise can also be an important component in a weight-reduction program (although not the primary one, which is diet).
- Obesity: While Americans have a new awareness about the benefits of eating a diet that promotes heart health, that positive trend is diminished by the extraordinary rise in obesity in the United States and increasingly worldwide. Today, 40 percent of Americans are clinically obese, or significantly overweight. Perhaps even more alarming, one in six children are now considered obese, and new research conducted over generations

clearly indicates that obese children are more likely to become obese adults. The connection between heart disease and obesity is multifaceted, because obesity increases your likelihood of developing many other risk factors for heart disease, including high blood pressure and diabetes. What remains clear is the strong correlation between obesity and heart disease. Adults between ages forty and fifty-nine who are overweight or obese have a 21 to 85 percent higher risk of developing cardiovascular disease as compared with their normal-weight peers.

- Substance abuse: Substance abuse has become a nationwide health crisis in just one generation, causing the deaths of seventy thousand Americans in 2018—more than HIV/AIDS at its peak and more than gun violence or car accidents in 2018. Today, on average 130 Americans die of an opioid overdose every day. Just as we seemed to be getting a handle on one aspect of the opioid crisis—overdose deaths from prescription narcotic painkillers had begun to decline—another opioid drug was becoming popular. The illicit and recreational use of a cheap, synthetic version of fentanyl—a drug ten times more powerful than morphine, originally designed for use in surgical procedures—has increased 45 percent since 2017. Forgotten somewhat in the focus on the opioid epidemic is that America's favorite legal drug, alcohol, continues to kill more people than all other drugs combined— more than eighty thousand in 2018. And while progress has been made in reducing the rates of smoking, more than 42 million Americans (or one in five) continue to smoke, accounting for 480,000 smoking-related deaths in the United States in 2018. The connection between substance abuse and heart disease is multifaceted, with nicotine, drugs, and alcohol damaging the heart muscle and blood vessels directly as well as contributing to the bad effects of other risk factors, including poor diet, lack of exercise, and impaired sleep.

- Anxiety, stress, and impaired sleep: Recent epidemiological studies have shown that people who face many stressors—from those who survive natural disasters to those who work long hours— are more likely to develop atherosclerosis, the accumulation of fatty plaques inside the coronary arteries. In addition to fats and cholesterols, the plaques contain monocytes and neutrophils, immune cells that cause inflammation in the walls of blood vessels. Chronic stress may cause some people to drink too much alcohol, smoke more, or binge eat, all of which can increase blood pressure and damage artery walls. Impaired sleep conditions, including insomnia and sleep apnea (thought to affect as much as 40 percent of the adult population), often have the same bad health effects and share many of the same symptoms as stress and anxiety.

In summary, your overall propensity for silent heart disease and coronary heart disease involves a unique combination of factors that you inherited from your parents and choices you've made as an adult. There's much you can do to lower your risk factors, particularly when it comes to lifestyle choices. In the next section, Part III, we'll look at the array of medications and diagnostic techniques that can help you and your physician maximize your heart health.

Part III

TESTS AND TREATMENT

PART III: INTRODUCTION

In Part II, we reviewed the various risk factors associated with silent heart disease. Looking over the last three decades since I wrote my last book, *Preventing Silent Heart Disease*, I can say with certainty that the world has become a more dangerous place.

There are increased risk factors that we could have never anticipated—an obesity epidemic, an opioid crisis, an increasingly stressful world caused by a nationwide obsession with social media and the inability to untether ourselves from emails and text messaging (even if we were so inclined). "Metabolic syndrome" quite literally was not in our vocabulary when I wrote my previous book in 1989. It's a cold, hard fact that in 2018 the life expectancy of the average American declined from the previous year, a first in recent times. It's unlike anything we've seen in the last one hundred years. (You have to go back to the early twentieth century to find a decline in life expectancy in the United States, which was largely due to combat deaths during World War I and, most importantly, the devastating Spanish flu pandemic of 1918 to 1920.)

On the other hand, we have options for the detection, treatment, and prevention of silent heart disease that we could have never dreamed of thirty years ago: stem cell therapy, 3-D-printed organic tissue, new medications and surgical innovations tailored to specific aspects of cardiac disease, and amazing technology like implantable devices and incredibly accurate wearable health monitors (disguised as smartphones and watches).

All things considered, I remain optimistic. We have made real progress over the last six decades in combatting heart disease and the related condition of stroke, the two biggest causes of death in the United States (not to mention significant progress in treating the third-biggest cause of death, cancer). America's suddenly shrinking life expectancy stems from failure to detect earlier and treat not coronary heart disease but mainly three preventable causes of death: drug overdose, chronic liver disease (related to drug and alcohol abuse), and suicide.

In this next section of the book, we'll dive deep into the dazzling array of technology and pharmacology available to us in the very near future. But we'll begin Part III by reviewing the latest in medications, diagnostics, therapies, and surgical techniques available today.

15

DIAGNOSTIC TESTS

If you have one or more risk factors for coronary heart disease, your doctor is likely to recommend that you undergo one or more diagnostic tests beyond the basic physical exam (during which a medical professional measures your blood pressure, takes your pulse, and listens to your heart with a stethoscope). These additional cardiac tests can help determine if you may already have had a silent heart attack (the kind with no symptoms). Remember that about half of all persons with coronary heart disease have the asymptomatic version, or silent heart disease.

If it's determined you already have had a heart attack, the tests can also determine how much of your heart was damaged and also what degree of coronary artery disease you may have. The tests screen your heart and help the doctor determine what treatment and lifestyle changes will help keep your heart healthy and prevent serious future medical events.

If that sounds scary, it shouldn't. Most cardiac tests today are non-invasive or minimally invasive. There are scores of cardiac tests available today, and in this chapter we'll review the most widely used ones.

ELECTROCARDIOGRAM (EKG) AND HOLTER MONITORING

Perhaps nothing better illustrates how far cardiac diagnostic testing has come than the history of the Holter monitor, whose origins harken back to the 1930s. That's when physicist Norman J. Holter began his pioneering studies in the electric potentials of muscles, nerves, and brain waves. The rapid advancements in electronic technology in the early twentieth century, such as the cathode ray oscilloscope (the same technology used in TV sets and computer monitors before the advent of flat screens) and other innovations developed during World War II, enabled the design of a system for sending electrical impulses from the human body through the air to a recorder.

Holter's device marked the beginning of radio-electrocardiography. Previously, cardiologists were limited to examining a patient's heart with the standard electrocardiogram for a one-minute period, during which time they might have sixty to seventy heartbeats to review. Holter's device permitted an evaluation of up to ten hours of heart action, and because the device was portable, the measurements could be taken in real-world circumstances, like a patient's home or workplace, not just in the physician's office or a researcher's laboratory. As a result, for the first time, measurement of the effects of the stress of ordinary life and work activities on heart action provided a much more accurate evaluation of cardiac health.

It was a miracle! Nevertheless, the first Holter "portable" devices weighed eighty-five pounds, and the first patients to use them literally had to wear a backpack to carry them. The invention of the transistor in 1952 permitted miniaturization of the early transmission equipment into a relatively light, four-pound recording device. The need for NASA to measure astronauts' vital functions in space further refined and miniaturized the equipment. Fast-forward to the twenty-first century and today's version of the Holter, which only weighs four ounces and can be worn around the neck on a chain. Competing cardiac monitors, or ambulatory electrocardiography devices, include the popular Zio, which is the size of a Band-Aid and is applied to the skin in the same way, with no loose wires or batteries to charge.

On a personal note, the Holter device was instrumental in my first published findings on silent heart disease fifty years ago. My research colleagues and I analyzed literally tens of thousands of magnetic tapes, which was how Holter devices recorded patients' electrocardiograms at the time, to help formulate our underlying theory that reduced blood flow to the heart (ischemia) could occur without pain. Our findings were published in a paper titled "Clinical Applications of Dynamic Cardiography," but in retrospect perhaps we should have simply called it, "Thank you, Dr. Holter."

Today's cardiac monitor devices essentially perform the same function as the early Holter devices—recording the electrical activity of the heart during daily activities. In developing your cardiac risk profile, your doctor may ask you to wear a monitor to see if you have an arrhythmia —that is, a slow, fast, or irregular (uneven) heartbeat. Or your doctor may use it to see how well your medicines are working to treat these problems. If you have a pacemaker and feel dizzy, a monitor could determine if your pacemaker is working properly.

The monitors pose no risk, and wearing one isn't painful. You can carry the monitor in a pocket or pouch, slung across your shoulders or worn around your neck like a purse or camera, or attached to your belt. You can perform all your usual activities while you wear the monitor with these exceptions: don't bathe, shower, swim, or have X-rays while wearing the monitor, and stay away from high-voltage arc metal detectors or large magnets.

A technician will teach you how to keep a diary of your activities and symptoms during the test. It's important to keep an accurate diary. If you feel symptoms such as chest pain, shortness of breath, uneven heartbeats, or dizziness, note in your diary the time of day they began, how long they lasted, and what you were doing at the time. Your diary will be compared to the changes in your EKG recorded by the Holter monitor.

Now, your doctor may deem your wearing a portable cardiac monitor unnecessary and conduct an electrocardiogram in the office for a onetime measurement. Whether done via portable monitor or in the office, the test measures the same thing, recording the electrical activity of the heart, including the timing and duration of each electrical phase of your heartbeat.

With each beat, an electrical impulse (or "wave") travels through the heart. This wave causes the heart muscle to squeeze and pump blood from the heart. An EKG will show the timing of the heart's upper and lower chambers. The right and left atria, or upper chambers, make the first wave, called a "P wave." The line flattens while the electrical impulse goes to the bottom chambers. The right and left bottom chambers, or ventricles, make the next wave, called a "QRS complex." The final wave, or "T wave," represents electrical recovery, or return to a resting state for the ventricles.

An EKG gives two major kinds of information. First, by measuring time intervals on the EKG, a doctor can determine how long the electrical wave takes to pass through the heart. Finding out how long a wave takes to travel from one part of the heart to the next shows if the electrical activity is normal or slow, fast or irregular. Second, by measuring the amount of electrical activity passing through the heart muscle, a doctor may be able to find out if parts of the heart are too large, are overworked, or are not working properly.

The goal for each type of EKG is also the same—to determine if there's an arrhythmia, to discover if a heart attack has occurred in the past or is presently occurring, and to help predict if a heart attack is developing by monitoring changes in heart rhythm and other functions of the EKG.

CHEST X-RAY

Using an X-ray, pictures are taken of the structure and organs inside your chest, like your heart, lungs, and blood vessels. They can show if there are signs of heart failure, including whether the heart is enlarged or fluid is accumulating in the lungs as a result of heart failure. However, a chest X-ray doesn't show the inside structures of the heart.

In this test, a technician positions the patient next to the X-ray film. An X-ray machine will be turned on for a fraction of a second. During this time, a small beam of X-rays passes through the chest and makes an image on special photographic film. Sometimes two pictures are taken—a front and side view. The X-ray film takes only a few minutes to develop. Sometimes your cardiologist needs more than just the front and side chest X-rays.

There's no pain involved, and the amount of radiation used in a chest X-ray is very small—one-fifth the dose a person gets each year from natural sources, such as the sun and the ground. While this small amount of radiation isn't considered dangerous, the levels of exposure for a given test need to be considered in the context of other radiation-utilizing tests that may be part of the cardiac diagnosis, since the possible cumulative effects of repeated radiation exposure are of concern. However, pregnant women should avoid even this low level of radiation whenever possible.

ECHOCARDIOGRAM

This is a common test in which a handheld device, placed on the chest, uses high-frequency sound waves (ultrasound) to produce images of your heart's size, structure, and motion. It helps your doctor check if there are any problems with your heart's valves and chambers and to see how strongly your heart pumps blood. An echocardiogram performed before and after exercise is also used to detect areas of the heart where the blood supply through the coronary arteries to the heart muscle is reduced (see "exercise stress test" below).

CARDIAC COMPUTED TOMOGRAPHY

Also known commonly as a CT or CAT scan, computer imaging (tomography) refers to several noninvasive diagnostic imaging tests that use computer-aided techniques to gather images of the heart. A computer creates a three-dimensional image of the heart's chambers and coronary arteries supplying blood to the heart. It can show blockages caused by calcium deposits in the coronary arteries.

When contrast dye (iodine) is given during the scan, the test can be used to show blockages in the heart arteries. This is useful in patients with chest discomfort to see if the discomfort comes from lack of blood flow to the heart muscle caused by blocked heart arteries (angina). If the heart arteries are normal, the doctor can confidently look into other causes of chest pain that aren't related to the heart. A CT scan can also be used to check if coronary artery bypass grafts remain open, check for congenital heart defects (problems present at birth), and also check how the ventricles are working.

EXERCISE STRESS TEST

In this test, also known as treadmill or exercise cardiac stress test, a monitor with electrodes is attached to the skin on the chest area to record your heart function while you walk and/or run in place on a treadmill. Many aspects of your heart function can be checked, including heart rate, breathing, blood pressure, EKG, and how tired you become when exercising. It also can help determine your safe level of exercise and helps predict dangerous heart-related conditions such as angina pectoris (chest pain) or heart attack.

MRI

In a magnetic resonance imaging (MRI) test, you lie on a table inside a long tubelike machine that produces a magnetic field, which aligns atomic particles in some of your cells. Radio waves are broadcast toward these aligned particles, producing signals that create 3-D images of your heart.

BLOOD TESTS

When your heart muscle has been damaged, as in a heart attack, your body releases substances into your blood. Blood tests can measure the levels of these substances and show if, and how much of, your heart has been damaged.

A common test after a heart attack checks the level of troponin in your blood. Troponin is a group of proteins found in cardiac muscle fibers that regulate muscular contraction. Increased troponin levels occur when the heart muscle is strained or during the course of an acute heart attack.

Blood tests are also done to measure the level of other substances in your blood, such as blood fats (e.g., cholesterol and triglycerides) and minerals. For example, a blood test can measure levels of vitamin D, which is normally obtained via sunlight and foods such as mushrooms and fortified foods. A low vitamin D level has been associated with high blood pressure, arterial damage, congestive heart failure, poor brain health, and other important problems.

Another widely available blood test can measure Lipoprotein-a, or Lpa, an inherited form of low-density lipoprotein (LDL) bound to a special protein. Studies have shown a correlation between high levels of LDL and early cardiovascular disease.

Another blood test determines your level of ferritin, a protein in the blood that binds with iron. An iron overload can oxidize cells in the arteries, leading to heart disease, and can make blood more prone to clotting. Yet another blood test can measure uric acid. An elevated level is linked to cardiovascular damage and generalized cell membrane dysfunction.

As noted in Part II, a blood test can determine the level for a bio-marker for inflammation, which may occur during a heart attack. A high C-reactive protein level is usually a red flag that something in your life-style or health is amiss and should be eliminated or otherwise corrected.

Research over the last forty years has revealed that increased levels of homocysteine, an amino acid, may be associated with increased risk of vascular damage. A safe homocysteine level, as determined by a blood test, is under ten micromoles per liter, and patients with high levels can be treated with B complex vitamins, which is a pretty simple solution.

MORE CARDIAC TESTS

Beyond these commonly used tests, your cardiologist today has an arsenal of more specialized cardiac diagnostic tools. Here's a quick run-down of some the most widely used of them:

- Advanced cholesterol panel: Two people with an LDL level of 100 mg/dL can have different heart disease risks because it's pos-sible that they have widely different particle numbers and sizes. An advanced cholesterol panel blood test can tell you more about your LDL particle number and size, which may yield important clues to silent signs of clogged arteries.
- Carotid intimal medial thickness (CIMT) test: This exam uses an ultrasound machine to see inside the major carotid artery in the neck, which connects the heart to the brain. The ultrasound shows the thickness of the inner two linings of the wall of the artery (if these walls are getting too thick, it's a sign of early atherosclerosis). This test has received a high recommendation from the American College of Cardiology, and more than five hundred scientific studies speak to its effectiveness.

- Endopat: Healthy arteries spring back quickly after being squeezed, for example, by a blood pressure cuff. When blood vessels don't spring back, it is a sign of diseased arteries. When Mayo Clinic researchers did this test on more than 250 people and tracked their health for six years, those with poor blood flow had a higher risk of heart attack or death. Note: It's possible to have full-blown coronary artery disease (and even to have undergone bypass surgery or stenting) and still have normal artery function.
- Cardiac catheterization: This test examines the inside of your heart's blood vessels using a special X-ray imaging technique called angiography. A thin hollow tube called a catheter is threaded through a blood vessel in the arm, groin, or neck to the heart. Dye is injected from the catheter into blood vessels to make them visible by X-ray. This test is also particularly helpful in evaluating chest pain to show if plaque is narrowing or blocking coronary arteries and in measuring blood pressure within the heart and the amount of oxygen in the blood.

CLASSIFYING HEART HEALTH

Which cardiac tests are best for you will be decided by you and your doctors. However, doctors do follow sets of general guidelines that classify your condition to identify your risk factors and begin early, more aggressive treatment to help prevent heart attacks or heart failure. The two systems used to classify cardiac failure are these:

- New York Heart Association classification. This symptom-based scale classifies heart failure into four categories. In Class I heart failure, you don't have any symptoms. In Class II heart failure, you can perform everyday activities without difficulty but become winded or fatigued when you exert yourself. With Class III, you'll have trouble completing everyday activities. Class IV is the most severe, leaving you short of breath even at rest.
- American College of Cardiology/American Heart Association guidelines. This stage-based classification system uses letters *A* to *D*. The system includes a category for people who are at risk

of developing heart failure. For example, a person who has several risk factors for, but no signs or symptoms of, heart failure is designated as Stage A. A person who has heart disease but no common symptoms of heart failure, such as fatigue or shortness of breath, is designated as Stage B. Someone who has heart disease and is experiencing or has experienced signs or symptoms of heart failure is designated as Stage C, and a person with advanced heart failure requiring specialized treatments is designated as Stage D.

These scoring systems are not independent of each other, and your doctor might use them together to help determine your most appropriate treatment options. Once your tests are complete, your doctor can help you interpret your score and plan your treatment based on your condition.

16

TREATMENTS

If you've been diagnosed with silent heart disease or coronary heart disease or have experienced a heart attack or another heart event, your treatment will most likely include one or more medications that you may take for the rest of your life.

Medications, along with lifestyle changes, are the most common form of treatment for cardiovascular diseases. Hundreds of drugs have been developed over the last five decades for the treatment of heart patients. There are many ways to classify these medications, but for our purposes, we will categorize these drugs according to the four main cardiac problems they are designed to treat:

1. Cholesterol
2. Blood clots
3. Blood pressure
4. Chest pain

Every heart patient is different, so you'll need to work with your physician to create a regimen of medications specific to your condition. For example, you may take drugs to lower your cholesterol and manage your blood pressure but not for blood clots or chest pain. Your best friend or spouse could have another diagnosis and need another category of drug or perhaps three or all four of them.

Heart disease is not the same for everyone, so it may be treated differently in each individual. As a patient, expect your physician to adjust dosages of your medication(s) to find the right level for you and to minimize side effects. Coronary heart disease is a chronic disease; there is no cure for it. However, much can be done to delay or limit its progression and to treat symptoms and complications. So, it's important to never stop taking a medication and never change your dosage or frequency without first consulting your doctor.

In the following discussion of the various types of medications, I will list their generic names followed in parentheses by their commercial brand names. We'll conclude this chapter with a discussion of other cardiac treatments beyond pharmaceuticals, notably surgical options and implantable devices.

CHOLESTEROL-LOWERING DRUGS

High cholesterol levels in your blood can cause atherosclerotic plaque to build up and lead to narrowed or blocked blood vessels. This is one of the leading causes of heart attack, stroke, and other serious heart problems. Cholesterol medications help lower your levels of low-density lipoprotein (LDL), or "bad" cholesterol, and raise your levels of high-density lipoprotein (HDL), or "good" cholesterol.

Statins are the most widely used drugs to lower bad cholesterol. Since their introduction in 1987, statins have evolved into seven different kinds for patients to use, depending on their needs. Generally statins are effective in lowering cholesterol levels by 20 to 60 percent, as well as reducing cardiovascular inflammation. Most people who have had a heart attack or stroke, bypass surgery, stents, or diabetes should be taking statins, as should patients with a high LDL level with or without heart disease. Some physicians prescribe statins for patients with multiple risk factors (e.g., advanced age, poor diet, sedentary lifestyle) to try to prevent the progression or onset of coronary heart disease with or without symptoms.

Common types of statin drugs are atorvastatin (Lipitor), pravastatin sodium (Pravachol), and simvastatin (Zocor). While statins remain the drug of choice for most physicians, there are other kinds of drugs that can lower cholesterol for patients who might be allergic to statins, including bile acid resins such as cholestyramine, cholesterol absorption inhibitors such as ezetimibe (Zetia), fibric acid derivatives such as fenofibrate (Tricor), and nicotinic acid such as niacin (Niacor), although these drugs tend to be less effective in lowering cholesterol levels.

BLOOD THINNERS (ANTICOAGULANTS)

In addition to a statin, your doctor may prescribe a drug to prevent a buildup of plaque in the blood vessels. The buildup of plaque can lead to blood clots, which in turn can cause serious problems when they break free of the plaque and partly or completely block blood flow to the heart and cause a heart attack. If the blood clot travels to the lungs, a pulmonary embolism could result. And if a clot travels to the brain, a stroke could occur.

While colloquially knowns as blood thinners, it's important to note that anticoagulants don't actually make the blood less concentrated or dissolve existing blood clots. Anticoagulants work by preventing blood clots from forming. Some do this by preventing your body from making substances called clotting factors. Others keep the clotting factors from working or prevent other chemicals from forming so that clots can't develop.

Aspirin, one of the oldest drugs known, is an over the counter anticoagulant used by millions of Americans for its painkilling effects. The ancients used as a painkiller the extract of willow bark—which naturally contains the anti-inflammatory ingredient salicin, a chemical component of modern-day aspirin. The synthesized form of the active chemical ingredient in aspirin, acetylsalicylic acid, was developed and first marketing by the Bayer pharmaceutical company in 1899. Its cardiovascular benefits were discovered in the 1960s. Aspirin can help to keep arteries open because of its anticlotting and antiplatelet effects. A standard dosage for heart patients is eighty-one milligrams per day, which is one baby aspirin. Aspirin makes sense for people who already have heart disease but not necessarily for people who just have risk factors, although many patients with high-risk profiles take daily aspirin preventively. Examples of other anticoagulants are enoxaparin (Lovenox), heparin (many brand names, including Fragmin and Lovenox), and warfarin (Coumadin).

Like anticoagulants, antiplatelet medications help prevent blood clots, but they work in a different way by preventing your body from making a substance, called thromboxane, that tells platelets to stick together to form a clot. Antiplatelet medicines include clopidogrel (Plavix), prasugrel (Effient), and ticagrelor (Brilique). They are prescribed with, or instead of, aspirin by some physicians.

You usually need antiplatelet medicines if you've had coronary angioplasty and stent implantation or have had recurring heart attacks or angina. Aspirin is both an anticoagulant and an antiplatelet drug. Other leading antiplatelet drugs are clopidogrel (Plavix) and prasurgel (Effient).

DRUGS FOR LOWERING BLOOD PRESSURE

As we learned earlier, one in three Americans suffers from hypertension or high blood pressure, a leading cause of silent heart disease and coronary heart disease. Well over thirty drugs or drug combinations are available for the treatment of elevated blood pressure.

ACE (angiotensin converting enzyme) inhibitors have been used for the treatment of hypertension for more than twenty years. They lower blood pressure by altering a biological control mechanism, the renin-angiotensin system. Renin is a hormone-like material produced by the kidneys that stimulates the production of angiotensin, a substance that tends to elevate blood pressure. ACE inhibitors lower the blood pressure by "inhibiting," or blocking, the actions of angiotensin. Examples of these drugs are captopril (Capoten), enalapril (Vasotec), lisinopril (Zestril, Prinivil), benazepril (Lotensin), and ramipril (Altace).

For those individuals who are unable to tolerate the ACE inhibitors, an alternative group of drugs, called angiotensin receptor blockers (ARBs), may be used. These drugs act on the same hormonal pathway as ACE inhibitors but instead block the action of angiotensin II at its receptor site directly. A small, early study of one of these agents suggested a greater survival benefit in elderly congestive heart failure patients as compared to an ACE inhibitor. However, a larger follow-up study failed to demonstrate the superiority of ARBs over ACE inhibitors. Further studies are underway to explore the use of these agents in congestive heart failure both alone and in combination with ACE inhibitors. Commonly prescribed ARBs are candesartan (Atacand), eprosartan (Teveten), irbesartan (Avapro), losartan (Cozaar), telmisartan (Micardis), and valsartan (Diovan).

Beta-blockers, which belong to the class of drugs that act upon nerve receptors, also can be useful in the treatment of high blood pressure. Beta-blockers can slow your heartbeat and lower your blood pressure and risk of a heart attack. You may sometimes be given a beta-blocker for arrhythmias (abnormal heart rhythms) or angina (see below).

This class of drugs not only slows your heart rate and reduces blood pressure but also limits or reverses some of the damage to your heart if you have systolic heart failure. Beta-blockers may reduce signs and symptoms of heart failure, improve heart function, and help you live longer. Commonly prescribed beta-blockers include acebutolol (Sectral), atenolol (Tenormin), betaxolol (Kerlone), bisoprolol/hydrochlorothiazide (Ziac), bisoprolol (Zebeta), metoprolol (Lopressor, Toprol XL), nadolol (Corgard), propranolol (Inderal), and sotalol (Betapace).

Vasodilators are another class of drugs found to be very effective in controlling blood pressure. These drugs "dilate," or open, the peripheral blood vessels. Initially, the vasodilators most widely used were hydralazine (Apresoline) and minoxidil (Rogaine—yes, the same drug used as a topical ointment to promote hair growth), but in recent years a new class of drugs, called calcium channel blockers, have been found to be particularly effective in treating not only high blood pressure but also problems associated with silent heart disease and coronary heart disease. Calcium is needed for all muscles to move, including the heart. Calcium channel blockers work by regulating the amount of calcium that enters muscle cells in your heart and blood vessels. This makes your heart beat less forcefully and helps blood vessels relax.

Your doctor may prescribe a calcium channel blocker if you have high blood pressure, chest pain, or a heart arrhythmia. Commonly prescribed calcium channel blockers include amlodipine (Norvasc), diltiazem (Cardizem), and nifedipine (Procardia).

DRUGS FOR MANAGING ANGINA

Angina pectoris literally means "choking in the chest." Earlier, we learned that symptom-free, high-risk patients with silent heart disease may have a much higher mortality rate from heart attacks and sudden death than other patients with coronary heart disease. Patients who have previously suffered angina and a heart attack and also have a history of silent heart disease are at very high risk for a recurrent heart attack and even death. In short, the successful management of angina is a matter of life and death for anyone but especially those who have suffered silent heart disease in the past.

Among the most widely prescribed antianginal medicines are nitrates, which have been used in one form or another since 1867. They act by relaxing the muscular walls of both arteries and veins, thereby (1) opening up the coronary arteries and permitting more oxygen-rich blood to flow to the heart muscle itself, and (2) dilating arteries in the periphery (the arms and legs), diminishing the amount of work done by the heart and reducing its oxygen requirements. Nitroglycerine, a rapidly acting nitrate administered under the tongue, is the treatment of choice for acute anginal chest pains. (This is the one of the drugs you're likely to get at an ER if you're experiencing chest pains.) Nitrates reduce both symptomatic and symptom-free episodes of inadequate coronary blood flow (ischemia). Intravenous nitroglycerine infusions are used to eliminate all episodes of silent heart disease. Some commonly prescribed forms of nitrates are isosorbide dinitrate (Dilatrate-SR, Isordil), isosorbide mononitrate (ISMO), and nitroglycerin (Nitro-Dur, Nitrolingual, Nitrostat).

Beta-blockers and calcium channel blockers are also used to treat angina.

BEST DRUG COMBINATIONS

Now, earlier in the chapter, I explained how cardiac treatment is highly individualized. What works for Jane might not work for Joe or June, John or Janice. Still, that doesn't mean research hasn't been conducted on what combination of cardiac medications is the best on average.

Researchers from the William Harvey Research Institute at Queen Mary University of London in the United Kingdom recently conducted a large long-term study that looked at the efficacy of different treatments in keeping cardiovascular disease at bay. The question that they hoped to answer in the Anglo-Scandinavian Cardiovascular Outcomes Trial was, Which treatments work best for preventing cardiovascular events?

Their test subjects were 8,580 UK participants who had high blood pressure as well as several risk factors for developing cardiovascular disease. One group received "traditional" treatment with a blood pressure drug and a diuretic, which is a drug often prescribed for high blood pressure. A diuretic increases the amount of water and salt expelled from the body as urine, which in turn decreases the amount of fluid flowing through the blood vessels, reducing pressure on the vessel walls. The other group received an "innovative" treatment consisting of a blood pressure drug and a statin (the go-to drug for lowering cholesterol).

The results, published in 2018, were unequivocal: the group receiving the innovative treatment had markedly better cardiovascular health. In fact, the new treatment was so successful that the study was stopped midstream. So many more lives were being saved with the new protocol that the researchers in good conscience could not continue with the traditional treatment. In fact, after five years with the new treatment, the subjects had on average nearly a 30 percent better chance of not succumbing to fatal heart disease.

While previous studies had shown that statins conferred long-term survival benefits, this study was among the first to confirm the importance of a regimen that aims to lower blood pressure and cholesterol together. Since high blood pressure and high cholesterol are two of the most common risk factors for silent heart disease, the findings could be relevant to tens of millions of Americans.

BEYOND MEDICATIONS

For most patients diagnosed with coronary heart disease, including silent heart disease, treatment will consist of one or more medications. However, in some instances, their doctors might recommend surgery to treat an underlying problem that led to heart symptoms. Among the surgical options are those required to implant devices in selected cases. The following are some of the most widely used procedures.

- Coronary bypass surgery: This procedure is meant to correct severely narrowed or completely blocked coronary arteries. It's the most common type of heart surgery, with more than two hundred thousand operations performed annually in the United States.
- Heart valve repair or replacement: If a faulty heart valve is causing your heart failure, your doctor may recommend repairing or replacing the valve to eliminate backward blood flow. Surgeons

can also repair the valve by reconnecting valve leaflets, by removing excess valve tissue so that the leaflets can close tightly, or by tightening or replacing the ring around the valve (annuloplasty). Once requiring open-heart surgery, today certain types of heart valve repair or replacement can be done with either minimally invasive surgery or by using cardiac catheterization techniques.

- Implantation of a cardioverter-defibrillator: An implantable cardioverter-defibrillator (ICD) is a device similar to a pacemaker, which is implanted under the skin of the chest with wires leading through the veins to the heart. If your heart starts beating at a dangerous rhythm or stops, the ICD is designed to shock it back into normal rhythm. An ICD can also function as a pacemaker and speed your heart up if it is going too slow.

- Cardiac resynchronization therapy (CRT) or biventricular pacing: A device is implanted next to the heart to send timed electrical impulses to both of the heart's lower chambers (the left and right ventricles), so that they pump in a more efficient, coordinated manner, thus preventing heart failure from worsening. Often the CRT is combined with an ICD.

- Implantation of a ventricular assist device (VAD): This implantable mechanical pump, which is attached to a failing heart muscle, facilitates the pumping of blood from the lower chambers of the heart (the ventricles) to the rest of the body. This device is often used in lieu of heart transplant surgery. About thirty-five hundred VADs are implanted in patients every year.

- Heart transplant: Some people have such severe heart failure that surgery or medications don't help enough, and they will need their compromised heart replaced with a healthy donor heart. The most common reason is that one or both ventricles are no longer functioning properly, and severe heart failure is present. Once a rare and exotic procedure, today approximately thirty-five hundred heart transplants are performed every year around the world, more than half of them in the United States. Still, because of the complexity of the surgery and the long wait time required for a donor heart, this is usually the procedure of last resort. There's no question that remarkable progress has been made since the first human heart transplant was performed more a half century ago by Dr. Christiaan Barnard. Today, the National Institutes of Health estimate that the procedure extends the average heart transplant patient's life by ten years.

In the next chapter, we'll get a preview of what medical science already has planned for the new generation of diagnostics and treatments.

17

HEART DISEASE IN THE
TWENTY-FIRST CENTURY

Imagine a twenty-first century in which the deadliest scourge of humankind, heart disease—which in 2019 alone killed an American every thirty-eight seconds and cost the health-care system more than $555 billion—has been conquered. The disease would still exist but would have been tamed, just like tuberculosis was at beginning of the twentieth century, polio by the mid-twentieth century, and HIV/AIDS at the beginning of the twenty-first century. In this case, it wouldn't be a vaccine or serum that eliminated heart disease as the leading killer of adults but rather a collection of clinical hardware, artificial intelligence (AI) software and Big Data, biological innovations, digital therapeutics, gene mapping, miniature implants, continuous-monitoring wearable devices, and bioprinted artificial heart tissue.

In this new world with greatly diminished deaths from heart disease, you would receive medications tailored to your own genetic profile to prevent the symptoms. A chatbot (think Siri) would remind you when to take your medications and also provide the latest findings of research relevant to your specific heart condition. But you really wouldn't have to worry as much about a heart condition anymore because if you were prone to one—through familial or environmental factors—you already would have been prescreened with biomarker testing, genetic polygenic risk assessments, advanced computer imaging systems, and algorithmic identifiers to give optimal management and treatment strategies. For example, if your condition involved an irregular heartbeat (arrhythmia), you might have had a microscopic, wireless implant inserted next to your heart to provide the appropriate electric signal, which then could be monitored continuously by your own or your physician's smartphone. If your heart was already damaged, a new valve or artery would be imprinted using engineered organic materials or harvested from off-the-shelf, allogenic stem cells. Cholesterol levels too high? You would be injected with nanoparticles that would whisk away the bad cholesterol and deliver it to the liver, where it could be broken down naturally. And your overall risk factors for chronic diseases, including heart disease and diabetes (a leading risk factor of heart disease), would be mitigated with drugs that target and block inflammation (if that is the main problem).

In short, this next era of heart disease treatment will not only slow the course of heart disease but be able to reverse any damage already done. In this chapter, we'll take a glimpse of the future—that is, the near future, because everything about to be discussed is already in some stage of research or development.

NEXT-GENERATION DIAGNOSTICS

Technology for the detection of heart disease is of exponentially increasing value. One of the most promising areas combines traditional diagnostics with cutting-edge artificial intelligence. Futurists say we're at the dawn of the fourth "industrial revolution," or breakthrough in technology. If steam power and electricity were at the center of the first two industrial revolutions, then we're currently in the third, dominated by electronics and digital technology. But it's the fourth revolution—the seamless synthesis of technologies, blurring the lines between technology, biology, and information—that holds the great potential for taking medicine to the next level. Artificial intelligence is key to the promise of the fourth revolution for heart disease detection and treatment.

What is artificial intelligence? It's defined as the ability of computer systems to perform human tasks. Essentially, programmable machines learn for themselves. Robotics are part of the AI revolution but are more important in manufacturing. For medicine, the most important aspects are algorithms (mathematical rules and models) and how they integrate into computer systems. In short, AI allows us mortal humans to perform herculean informational tasks and calculations not previously possible.

Verily is an example of an artificial intelligence algorithm. Designed by researchers from Google and its health-tech subsidiary, it promises to predict heart disease just by taking one glance at a patient's eyes. To build this technology, scientists scanned a database of nearly three hundred thousand patients for patterns. The "eye scans" evaluate the networks of blood vessels in the interior wall of the eye, revealing telltale signs of heart disease, such as high blood pressure. Although still in the testing stage, it's believed the eye scan will be able to predict with 70 percent accuracy whether a patient will suffer a heart issue in the next five years.

Wearable devices are another area of new diagnostic technology. You might say that the first "wearable" in cardiovascular medicine dates back to the 1800s, when a watch with a second hand was used to measure heart rate. Today, however, wearables can monitor everything from heart rate and rhythm to blood pressure, sleep quality and duration, and physical activity. In 2018 Apple introduced its Apple Watch series featuring an electrocardiogram (EKG) function that measures heartbeat and detects irregular rhythms. Wearers are alerted with a notification if they are experiencing atrial fibrillation (an abnormal heart rhythm).

Two apps now available that I think are especially useful are Instant Heart Rate, which turns your phone's camera lens into a heart rate monitor, recording your beats per minute, and Smart Blood Pressure, which allows you to take blood pressure readings wherever and whenever. (No more needing to visit the doctor's office or pharmacy for a pressure cuff.)

Another smartphone app, which has been developed by researchers at the Indian Institute of Technology Bombay, will be able to detect heart attacks up to six months beforehand by measuring a cardiac biomarker. Specifically, it measures myoglobin, an iron-containing protein released into the bloodstream soon after myocardial infarction, or the sudden blockage of blood flow to the heart that leads to a heart attack.

There's another diagnostic heart tool that's among the most promising, however, as the headline in a recent article in the Johns Hopkins newsletter article declared, *coronary artery calcium score* is "The Heart Test You Might Need—but Likely Haven't Heard of." Why is this important, potentially life-saving diagnostic tool under the radar? One answer is that many insurance companies still won't pay for it. Like tests for cholesterol, blood pressure, and blood sugar, coronary artery calcium (CAC) testing helps reveal your risk of heart disease but often before other diagnostic tests. The test is painless and quick. A CT scan takes

images of your heart and coronary arteries that may show specks of calcium called calcifications—early signs of coronary artery disease.

Using data from almost seven thousand subjects, Johns Hopkins
researchers compared two approaches to calculating heart risk. One way
used only the traditional risk factors, like smoking, cholesterol, blood
pressure, and diabetes. The other included the coronary calcium scan
score. Results reported in the *European Heart Journal* showed that by
looking at the coronary calcium scan, doctors could much better estimate heart disease risk, especially for those thought to be at low risk or
high risk. Fifteen percent of those thought to be at very low risk using
traditional risk factors actually had high coronary artery calcium scores.
And 35 percent of those thought to be at high risk showed no coronary
artery calcium and therefore had a lower risk of heart events. These
finds echoed those from a previous study by Emory University of 9,715
participants who showed no symptoms of coronary artery disease at the
time of the scans. Fifteen years later, researchers found the CAC scores
accurately predicted heart disease in the patients.

Another side of the fourth revolution in medicine is the advent
of Big Data. Analytics software combined with artificial intelligence is
allowing medical professionals to identify high-risk patients before they
become sick. Using data from large clinical trials conducted by studies
previously funded by the National Institutes of Health, University of
Texas Southwestern Medical Center researchers developed a way to
predict which patients would benefit most from proactive treatment of
high blood pressure. The algorithm they formulated combined three
measurements routinely collected during clinical visits and was able to
successfully identify a subgroup of patients who were at the highest risk
for early major adverse cardiovascular events, including heart attack,
stroke, and death (from a heart event). In effect, Big Data offers the
opportunity to conduct so-called retrospective clinical studies in which
new life is breathed into old research.

On the horizon in diagnostic and therapeutic tools is what's been
called "personalized prescribing." Already there are testing panels available that analyze your genes to determine your probable response to
medications commonly prescribed for attention deficit hyperactivity disorder and certain mental health disorders. Watch for this technology to
be refined so that it guides not only drug selection but individualized dos-

ing. At the moment, virtually all drugs are dispensed with dosages based on averages (and as discussed earlier in the book, usually with a bias toward males). Imagine soon selecting a cardiac medication that you know in advance will produce no or minimal side effects for your physiology and whose dosage is precisely customized for your individual genome.

In 2018 a novel imaging biomarker that can predict the risk of cardiac mortality was announced by a group of researchers led by Dr. Milind Desai from the Cleveland Clinic. Using Big Data collected from previous studies conducted between 2005 and 2009, the research showed conclusively that patients with significant coronary inflammation were associated with significantly higher rates of death from cardiac causes. The imaging biomarker, called the perivascular fat attenuation index, or FAI, revealed coronary inflammation by mapping the changes in perivascular fat. The diagnostic biomarker might prove transformative someday for prevention, because it's based on a routine test that is already used in everyday clinical practice but for the first time captures a cardiac risk factor currently missed by all other risk scores and noninvasive tests. Knowing who is at risk for a heart attack allows for earlier intervention.

Now, what if an individual's DNA sequence, or genome, could predict heart disease in people who have not yet had a heart attack or who might be at risk for silent heart disease? In a study whose findings were published in the *American Heart Journal* in 2019, researchers used polygenic risk scores (PRSs), which are based on an individual's entire genome sequence, to predict the risk of developing coronary artery disease. The study's finding confirmed earlier research that showed PRSs are an effective predictive tool in identifying people with a high risk for heart attack. The next step is to test the genetic scoring to determine if managing and treating people based on PRSs improves their heart health. The American Heart Association named the use of PRSs as one of the biggest advances in heart disease research in 2018.

NEW MEDICATIONS

The rapid pace of pharmacology continues unabated in cardiovascular medicine. In 2018 a record forty-six new drugs were approved by the Food and Drug Administration (FDA). Although statins remain the mainstay of lipid-lowering medications, the arsenal of pharmacotherapy for treatment of blood cholesterol has expanded to include PCSK9 inhibitors, the class of drugs that consumes the most attention among cardiologists. The enthusiasm for these biologic drugs within the medical community revolves around their capacity to reduce cardiac events in patients with known heart disease. PCSK9 inhibitors are proteins made in a laboratory. They target other proteins in your body, specifically your liver, which has cell receptors that sweep away excess cholesterol. But the PCSK9 protein actually destroys the cell receptors. That's where the "inhibitors" part come in. They latch onto PCSK9 proteins and block them from acting. The result: more receptors are able to do their job. This lowers the amount of low-density lipoprotein (LDL) cholesterol in your blood. In fact, one review of studies found that PCSK9 inhibitors slash LDL levels by an average of 47 percent, and the PCSK9 drugs were shown to reduce the risk of heart attacks by 27 percent.

It's estimated that 10 million Americans with high cholesterol could benefit from PCSK9 inhibitors. However, this promising new class of drugs faces two hurdles—cost and delivery. The PCSK9 drugs can cost as much as fifty times more than statins for a year's supply. Also, they're only available in an injectable form at the moment, which will discourage many patients from using them.

A drug is typically manufactured through chemical synthesis, which means that it is made by combining specific chemical ingredients in an ordered process. PCSK9 is a biologic drug, which is manufactured in a living system such as a microorganism or plant or animal cells. Many biologics are produced using recombinant DNA technology. Currently, available cardiovascular drugs with anti-inflammatory effects, such as aspirin and statins, predominantly exert therapeutic benefits by means other than inflammation suppression. While no definitive evidence has documented that reducing inflammation of the blood vessels will reduce cardiac events, this is a major focus of ongoing research. The research is part of a larger theory that inflammation could be the underlying cause of most chronic diseases—from diabetes to dementia, including coronary heart disease. Studies have indicated, for example, that a good deal of the benefit from exercise to cardiovascular health is attributable to its effect in lowering inflammation in the body.

A 2017 clinical trial called CANTOS involved another biologic drug, canakinumab, which blocks a specific pro-inflammatory pathway called IL-1beta. The findings were startling. This was the first scientifically gathered evidence that drugs that block inflammation could be the next chapter in cardiac medications. The trial, which involved more than ten thousand patients in thirty-nine countries, was primarily designed to determine whether an anti-inflammatory drug, by itself, could lower rates of cardiovascular disease in a large population, without simultaneously lowering levels of cholesterol, as statin drugs do. The answer was a definitive yes, and therefore the pharmaceutical industry is now deeply interested in finding ways to stop cardiac inflammation with medicines.

As we learned earlier, age is a primary risk factor in heart disease. So, what if you could turn back the clock with a medication that, in effect, slows down the heart's aging process? Researchers have discovered that relaxin, a reproductive hormone, can suppress cardiovascular disease symptoms. "A common problem in age-associated cardiovascular disease is altered electrical signaling required for proper heart contraction," explained Brian Martin, the lead researcher in a study on the therapeutic benefits of relaxin, in an article published in *Science Daily*. "When ions in the heart and their associated channels to enter or exit the heart are disrupted, complications occur." A relaxin medication might one day soon be given to patients of a certain age with a high-risk cardiac profile as part of regular cardiac therapy.

SURGICAL INNOVATIONS

Of course, the goal of any cardiologist is to avoid having a patient undergo surgery. A wise man once said that a good physician is one who successfully treats his patient; a great physician is one who prevents the patient from needing treatment in the first place. But in some cases the best solution to a heart problem is a surgical procedure. New surgical innovations are embracing minimally invasive procedures and new technologies, including robotics.

Harvard University and Boston Children's Hospital researchers came up with a soft robot that fits around the heart and helps it beat. The device holds much promise for individuals whose heart has been weakened by a heart attack and who are at risk of heart failure. The robot syncs with the heart through a thin silicone sleeve with soft pneumatic actuators that mimic the heart's outer muscle layers. It does so without any direct contact with the blood, as is the case with most currently available devices. This removes the need for potentially dangerous blood thinner medications.

Transcatheter aortic valve replacement (TAVR) is the replacement of the aortic valve of the heart through the blood vessels (as opposed to valve replacement by open-heart surgery). The replacement valve is delivered via one of several access points in the body (i.e., upper leg, collar bone, belly button). Until recently, surgical aortic valve replacement was the standard of care in adults with severe symptomatic aortic stenosis. However, since the risks associated with open-heart surgery are increased in elderly patients (and especially those who already have cardiovascular disease, chronic kidney disease, or chronic respiratory dysfunction), eliminating or reducing the risks of such surgery through new and minimally invasive procedures is certainly warranted. (The FDA recently approved TAVR.)

STEM CELLS AND BIOPRINTING

Stem cell and gene therapies and bioprinted tissue (using a 3-D printer) offer the prospect of creating new organic tissue to replace irreparably damaged heart tissue—the stuff of science fiction only a generation ago. Imagine replacing a damaged artery or valve or—wait for it!—the entire heart organ using one or both of these rapidly evolving procedures. This is the brave new world in the treatment of silent heart disease and the prevention of sudden death—a little scary because of possible unintended consequences but also irresistible for the potential to effectively treat heart conditions with a minimum of trauma.

BioCardia is one of a number of companies exploring biotechnology/regenerative medicine for the treatment of heart failure. Among its treatment modalities, personalized screenings help determine which patients are most likely to benefit from intramyocardial injection of therapeutic agents. BioCardia's current efforts in cardiac regenerative medicine include therapies that focus on heart failure resulting from heart attacks. The company was cofounded by Dr. Simon Stertzer, who performed the first coronary balloon angioplasty in the United States in 1978.

Can heart attack damage be reversed? Dr. Eduardo Marban of Cedars-Sinai Medical Center in Los Angeles is betting that it can. He recently launched a study using cells taken from the hearts of organ donors, avoiding altogether the need for a patient biopsy. Officially known as the Allogeneic Heart Stem Cells to Achieve Myocardial Regeneration (ALLSTAR) trial, the study aims to involve more than three hundred patients with moderate or severe heart damage. This is an ongoing study, but early results indicate that the amount of living heart muscle increased significantly, by 23 percent on average, in the test subjects.

Stem cell therapy is still new and finding its footing. The mechanism of how stem cells work and why they work as miraculous treatments for some but not for others is still unknown. In a recent article titled "Mending a Broken Heart: Stems Cells and Cardiac Repair," the National Institutes of Health noted that despite the relative infancy of this field, initial results from the application of stem cells to restore cardiac function have been promising.

Rather than growing replacement tissue for a damaged heart exclusively with stem cells, what if you could print it? Biolife4D, a Chicago-based biotech start-up, recently announced that it can "bioprint" a human cardiac muscle patch, using a patient's stem cells, which can be sutured over an area of dead heart muscle to speed up recovery from acute heart failure. In 2019, a group of Israeli researchers announced they had developed a 3-D-printed heart complete with a blood vessel system. The tissue was printed using fat tissue from a donor, as well as cells from the tissue that were cultured and reprogrammed into heart cells. The procedure marks the first time anyone anywhere has successfully engineered and printed an entire heart replete with cells, blood vessels, ventricles, and chambers. The technology could one day provide printed hearts for transplants that minimize rejection by a patient's immune system by using the patient's own cells.

IMPLANTABLE DEVICES AND BIONANOTECHNOLOGY

The problem with diagnostics that try to monitor a patient's heart condition is that they don't exist in the real world. What a patient's heart might reveal in a clinical setting when checked for a few minutes might differ entirely from what would be learned if it were monitored, say, around the clock for an entire week of the patient's everyday life. Until now, we've had to live with this issue—diagnostics machines were simply too big and bulky to be incorporated into the patients' real-world experience. Yes, wearable devices can provide the kind of data that only exists in the real world, but their downside is that they depend to a large degree on patient initiative. Even when patients follow instructions perfectly, there are times when the devices either can't be used (such as during bathing) or malfunction because of outside environmental factors ("Honey, the dog ate my wearable!").

All of that is about to change. Implantable devices offer the prospect of a shift from episodic testing to continuous monitoring without having to depend on patient compliance. Supported by artificial intelligence and software, these devices will allow for a minimizing of risk and optimization of intervention when treatment is necessary.

Similarly, bionanotechnology increasingly is being used in the diagnosis and treatment of cardiac diseases. Nanotechnology is a field of research and innovation concerned with building devices on the scale of atoms and molecules. (A nanometer is one-billionth of a meter, ten times the diameter of a hydrogen atom.) The medical application of this is known as bionanotechnology.

Nanoparticles have demonstrated potential in both detection and removal of atherosclerotic plaques, which causes the narrowing of coronary arteries. Nanoparticles can deliver therapeutic biomolecules to the site of coronary atherosclerosis and shrink plaques by reducing inflammation (for example, by activating pro-resolving pathways) and removing lipids and cholesterol crystals. And because nanoparticles can mimic or alter biological processes, they might someday soon be used to deliver medications over a prescribed period following an initial injection. Finally, nanoparticles could be an effective way to deliver stem cells and bioengineered tissue to repair cardiac damage.

PART III: TAKEAWAYS

W e're on the brink of a technological paradigm shift, the so-called fourth revolution of industrial development, that will fundamentally change how we detect and treat heart disease. Advances in artificial intelligence and Big Data, wearable and implantable devices, and the creation of organic replacement heart tissue through 3-D bioprinting and stem cell therapy will fuse seamlessly together to make the deadly specter of silent heart disease and coronary heart disease largely a thing of the past. These advances will not only prevent, or significantly delay the onset, of heart disease but, for the first time, allow for existing cardiac damage to be reversed.

In the meantime, we currently have an array of diagnostic tools, medications, and new surgical techniques that just a few years ago would have seemed futuristic. From CT scans to MRIs, today's diagnostics make the identification of cardiovascular problems more accurate than ever. The miniaturization of devices (EKGs) to continuously monitor the heart's electrical activity has revolutionized the evaluation of cardiac health.

If you are diagnosed with silent heart disease or coronary heart disease, today's medications provide your physician with an arsenal of time-tested drugs like cholesterol-lowering statins to scores of other pharmaceuticals for stopping blood clots, managing high blood pressure, and controlling angina (chest pain). Everyone's treatment regimen will be different; however, new research indicates that a majority of heart disease patients could benefit from a combination of a statin and, if needed, a drug to treat elevated blood pressure.

The vast majority of heart disease patients will primarily be treated with a regimen of lifestyle modifications and medications. Should your physician and you decide that surgery is the best treatment option, new techniques and implantable devices available now will significantly improve not only longevity but quality of life as well.

Part IV

RESOURCES

DIY CARDIAC RISK FACTOR TESTS

It's daunting to be reminded of the costs and consequences of heart disease:

- One in three deaths in the United States is due to cardiovascular disease, and about 160,000 occur in people under age sixty-five.
- One in every six health-care dollars is spent on cardiovascular disease.
- Heart disease kills more Americans each year than cancer, gun violence, and drug overdose combined.
- About 1.5 million heart attacks and strokes occur every year in the United States because of coronary heart disease.
- About half of those with heart failure will die within five years.
- About half of those who experience a heart attack have no previous symptoms (silent heart disease).

Here's the good news: most heart disease—including silent heart disease—is preventable, or can be significantly delayed, now! As we learned in Part II, risk factors such as high blood pressure and high cholesterol are easily manageable with modern-day medications. Another whole category of risk factors stem from lifestyle choices—how you eat, drink, exercise, and sleep.

The following two tests are designed to give you a quick snapshot of your cardiac risk factors. To be sure, they are not in any way a replacement for an evaluation by a medical professional, notably your doctor or cardiologist. However, the theme of this book is that knowledge is power, so the more you know about your cardiac health, the better.

The first is an online questionnaire developed by the American Heart Association, "Check. Change. Control. Calculator." You can access it here: https://ccccalculator.ccctracker.com.

The second, which follows, is an updated version of a quiz that I first created for my previous book, *Preventing Silent Heart Disease*.

If the results of the tests indicate you're at risk for heart disease—even moderate risk—consult with your doctor about a treatment regimen right for you.

CARDIAC RISK QUIZ

Answer the questions below as accurately as possible. (There are no "right" answers.) Note each question asks for the selection of one score. When you're finished, add all the scores and find your cardiac risk on the scale at the end of the quiz.

My age and sex:

0	woman younger than 50
+1	woman aged 50–65
+2	woman older than 65
+1	man younger than 40
+2	man aged 40–50
+3	man aged 50–65
+4	man older than 65

SCORE___

Among my parents or siblings, there have been heart problems (e.g., heart attacks, angina, sudden death) before the age of 60:

0	in no parent or sibling
+1	in 1 or more parents or siblings over the age of 60
+2	in 1 parent or sibling under the age of 60
+4	in 2 or more parents or siblings under the age of 60

SCORE___

Smoking (Tobacco Cigarettes)

0	I have never smoked

I quit smoking:

+1	over 5 years ago
+2	2–5 years ago
+3	1–2 years ago
+6	less than 1 year go

I now smoke:

+ 6	less than 10 cigarettes a day
+ 8	10–20 cigarettes a day
+16	20–40 cigarettes a day
+20	over 40 cigarettes a day

SCORE___

Cholesterol and Other Fats

My serum cholesterol level is

0	179 or less
+1	170–200
+2	200–240
+4	240–300
+6	over 300

SCORE___

My LDL is

0	130 or less
+2	131–160
+4	161–190
+6	over 190

SCORE___

My HDL is

0	over 60
+1	45–60
+2	30–44
+3	25–30
+4	less than 25

SCORE___

Blood Pressure

My blood pressure is
Age under 60

0	below 140/90
+4	140/90 or above

Age 60 or over

0	below 140/90
+1	between 140/90 and 180/96
+4	above 180/96

SCORE___

Diabetes

My fasting blood sugars have always been

0	normal
+1	occasionally elevated
+3	diabetes after age of 30
+4	diabetes before age of 30

SCORE___

Exercise

I exercise aerobically (running, vigorous walking, swimming, cycling, etc.)

0	regularly 3–5 times per week
+2	only on weekends
+4	little or none

SCORE___

Weight

My weight is

0	ideal
+1	5–10 percent overweight
+2	10–20 percent overweight
+3	20–30 percent overweight
+4	over 30 percent overweight

SCORE___

Stress

I feel stressed

0	rarely or not at all
+1	occasionally
+2	frequently
+4	all the time

SCORE___

TOTAL SCORE___

Your Cardiac Risk Factor

0–14 = low risk
14–24 = moderate risk
24 or more = high risk

EPILOGUE

A Final Word about Coronavirus

As I write this, the COVID-19 coronavirus—a virus similar to seasonal influenza but on a per capita basis more lethal—is sweeping the United States, with the full extent of its harm still being assessed. However, those of us living in North America do have the advantage of learning from how the pandemic emerged in China in January 2020 and its direct cardiovascular effects.

Here's what cardiologists on the frontline report, according to a clinical bulletin issued in mid-March 2020 by the American College of Cardiology:

- The majority of those actually hospitalized for the disease—by definition, the most serious cases—have one or more underlying chronic diseases, with 31 percent having hypertension and 14.5 percent having cardiovascular disease. (Some epidemiologists believe that one of the receptors involved in this virus is also associated with cardiovascular disease, but at the moment that's only a theory.)
- 10.5 percent of case fatalities occurred in patients with cardiovascular disease and 6 percent in patients with hypertension.
- Another 10 percent of those hospitalized for the virus also had diabetes, which as we learned in Chapter 9 is a common comorbidity of heart disease.

Bottom line: A good portion, perhaps as much as one-third, of cardiovascular patients in the United States are likely to get COVID-19 at some point. Those with cardiac injury from a previous event or an inherited heart condition appear to be particularly at risk. Even if you think that you currently don't have a cardiovascular disease but are at risk based on the information presented in this book, you should immediately consult your physician.

To be clear, COVID-19 could be with us for many more months. Not all coronaviruses are seasonal, and it will probably be a year or more before a vaccine is available.

How exactly COVID-19 affects the heart is not known yet, but likely it follows the same pattern of other viral infections that inflame the lungs and compromise oxygen intake. The good news, based on the preliminary data gathered in China as well as in Italy, is that most patients after recovering from COVID-19 will have normal heart function.

While it is still too early to say how to best treat cardiovascular patients who get COVID-19, a judicious use of high-intensity statins may be called for. Again, check with your physician or cardiologist, particularly in regards to the potential effect of high-statin usage on liver function.

Finally, this is a good time to remind all cardiovascular patients to a get a flu shot every fall before the start of flu season. A little over a majority of cardiovascular patients do get a flu shot, but that should be more on the order of 90 perecnt. While there is no vaccine yet for COVID-19, it's important to keep in mind that seasonal influenza to date has been far more deadlier over the past 12 months than COVID-19.

—Harold L. Karpman, MD, Los Angeles, March 2020

CARDIAC GLOSSARY

Acute   Having a rapid, intense onset and usually a short course with symptoms of varying degrees of intensity.

ACE inhibitors   A class of drugs that lower blood pressure by interfering with the body's production of angiotensin.

Adrenaline (epinephrine)   One of the hormones produced by the adrenal glands. It narrows the small blood vessels, increases the heart rate, and raises the blood pressure.

Aerobic exercise   A method of physical exercise for producing beneficial changes in the respiratory and circulatory systems by activities that require only a minimal or modest increase in oxygen intake.

Ambulatory ECG monitoring   See *Holter monitor* below.

Amphetamines   A class of drugs that stimulate the nervous system and suppress appetite.

Anaerobic exercise   A method of physical exercise in which more oxygen is used than is available, usually leading to exhaustion.

Aneurysm   A ballooning-out of the wall of a heart chamber or an artery blood vessel due to a weakening of the wall by disease, injury, or congenital defect.

Angina (angina pectoris)   Discomfort usually in the chest or in other locations (back, arm, neck, etc.) due to inadequate supply of blood and oxygen to the heart muscle, resulting from the narrowing or blockage of one or more coronary arteries.

Angiogram   Pictures of heart chambers or blood vessels taken during the course of an angiography examination. See *angiography*.

Angiography   An X-ray technique that involves the injection of dye, through a catheter, into the heart chambers or blood vessels, resulting in a detailed picture of the insides of these structures. See *angiogram*.

Angioplasty   A catheter technique to elevate and dilate narrowed coronary arteries at the point where they have become narrowed by plaque (see below).

Angiotensin converting enzyme inhibitors   See *ACE inhibitors*.

Antianginal drug   A drug used to relieve angina symptoms.

Antiarrhythmic drug   A drug that helps control or prevent cardiac arrhythmias.

Anticoagulants   Drugs, commonly called "blood thinners," that retard the blood-clotting process.

Antihypertensive   A drug that lowers blood pressure.

Aorta   The body's largest artery, which carries blood from the main pumping chamber (left ventricle) of the heart and distributes it to all parts of the body.

Aortic valve   The valve through which oxygenated blood passes from the main pumping chamber (left ventricle) of the heart to the body's largest artery. See *aorta*.

Arrhythmia   Any disturbance of the heart's normal rhythm.

Arterioles   The smallest arteries of the body, which conduct blood to the capillaries.

Arteriosclerosis   A disease of the lining of a coronary artery, which results in hardening and loss of elasticity of the arterial walls; commonly called "hardening of the arteries."

Arteriosclerotic heart disease   See *ischemic heart disease*.

Artery   A blood vessel that transports blood away from the heart to the rest of the body. An artery usually carries oxygenated blood, except in the case of the pulmonary artery, which carries unoxygenated blood from the heart to the lungs for a new oxygen supply.

Atheroma   A mass of yellowish fatty and cellular material that forms in and behind the inner lining of arterial walls.

Atherosclerosis   A form of arteriosclerosis in which, in addition to the hardening and loss of elasticity of the arteries, a fatty substance (plaque) forms on the inner walls of the arteries, frequently causing diminishment or obstruction of the flow of blood. See *arteriosclerosis*.

Atrium   One of the two upper chambers of the heart that receive unoxygenated blood from the body or lungs and transport it to the ventricles.

Atroventricular node   A small nodule of muscular fibers at the base of the wall behind the right and left atria that conducts impulses from the sinoatrial node to the ventricle.

Auscultation   The act of listening to sounds within the body, usually using a stethoscope.

Beta-blocker   A drug that blocks the action of the beta receptors, the nerve endings that affect the heart rate and force of contraction. Such drugs are used for the treatment and control of angina, high blood pressure, and certain cardiac arrhythmias.

Bile acid sequestrants   These medications (e.g., cholestyramine, colestipol) bind cholesterol-containing bile acids in the intestines and remove them in the feces.

Blood pressure   The force exerted by the blood against the arterial walls, created by the heart as it pumps blood to all parts of the body.

Blood vessel   A vein or artery.

Bradycardia   An abnormally slow heart rate, usually less than sixty beats per minute.

Bypass surgery   See *coronary artery bypass surgery.*

Calcium channel blocker   A drug that blocks the calcium transport mechanism in blood vessels and heart muscle cells. Such drugs relax the walls of the coronary arteries, preventing coronary spasm. They are used mainly for the treatment and prevention of angina.

Calorie   A numerical unit used to express the amount of heat output by an organism and the fuel or energy value of food.

Capillaries   Tiny, thin-walled blood vessels forming a network between the arterioles and the veins that facilitate the exchange of substances between the surrounding tissues and the blood.

Carbohydrate   One of the three food ingredients that supply energy to the body and are essential for normal body function.

Cardiac   Pertaining to the heart.

Cardiac arrest   Abrupt cessation of heartbeat.

Cardiac catheterization   See *catheterization.*

Cardiac cycle   One complete heartbeat, consisting of a contraction and a relaxation of the heart.

Cardiac output   The amount of blood pumped by the heart each minute.

Cardiologist   A physician specializing in the diagnosis and treatment of heart disease.

Cardiology   The study of the heart in health and disease.

Cardiomyopathy   A term for diseases of the heart muscle (myocardium), which can cause it to become stiff and weak.

Cardiopulmonary   Pertaining to the heart and lungs.

Cardiopulmonary resuscitation (CPR)   Emergency procedure for reviving heart and lung function, using special physical techniques and electrical and mechanical equipment.

Cardiovascular   Pertaining to the heart and blood vessels.

Cardioversion   The restoration of normal heart rhythm in patients afflicted with certain cardiac arrhythmias, after using an electric shock applied across the chest wall.

Catheter   A thin, flexible tube that, in cardiology, can be guided through a vein or artery (in the groin or arm) into the heart. It can be used to measure pressures, inject X-ray dye, or open up arteries.

Catheterization   In cardiology, the process of introducing a catheter into a vein or artery, then usually directing it toward the heart.

Cholesterol   A natural body fat found in foods of animal origin (meat, dairy products), but not in foods of plant origin; an ingredient in fatty plaques that may block coronary arteries. Blood cholesterol is made up of cholesterol manufactured in the liver and absorbed from ingested food.

Chronic   Of long duration or frequent recurrence.

Circulatory   Pertaining to the heart, blood vessels, and circulation.

Coagulation   The formation of a clot.

Collateral circulation   Circulation pathways using nearby smaller vessels going around a main artery that has been blocked.

Complex carbohydrates   Starch and fiber sugars from plants.

Congenital   Pertaining to an inherited feature; that which is present at birth.

Congestive heart failure   A condition in which a weakened heart is unable to pump enough blood, effectively leading to congestion of the lungs and retention of water in the body.

Constriction   A narrowing or tightening due to an inward pressure.

Contrast agent   An organic iodine solution that increases the radiodensity of blood so that the blood vessels will contrast with soft tissues of the heart and/or other tissues.

Coronary   Pertaining to the coronary arteries, the blood vessels that supply the heart muscle with blood and oxygen. Also, used as a noun, an abbreviated term for heart attack.

Coronary arteries   See *coronary*.

Coronary arteriogram   Pictures of coronary arteries taken with an X-ray technique involving injection of dye into the heart's blood vessels. See *angiography*.

Coronary artery bypass surgery   The surgical revascularization (see below) of the heart, using healthy blood vessels of the patient to bypass or circumvent obstructed coronary arteries and improve blood flow.

Coronary artery disease   Atherosclerosis of the coronary arteries. See *atherosclerosis*.

Coronary artery risk factor   See *risk factor*.

Coronary thrombosis   A blood clot in a coronary artery.

CT scan   In cardiology, a computer X-ray technique (computed tomography) for heart scanning.

Cyanosis   A bluish discoloration of the skin, fingernails, and lips due to insufficient oxygen in the blood. It is common in patients with certain types of congenital heart defects and other diseases.

Defibrillation   Termination of fibrillation (see below). Usually refers to the treatment of atrial or ventricular fibrillation (a life-threatening arrhythmia) by the application of an electric shock (cardioversion) and/or drugs.

Diabetes mellitus   A disorder of sugar metabolism characterized by inadequate production or utilization of the hormone insulin.

Diastole   The period of each heartbeat during which the pumping chambers (ventricles) relax and fill with blood.

Diastolic blood pressure   The diastolic reading obtained in blood pressure measurement (i.e., the second or lower number).

Dietary cholesterol   Cholesterol contained in ingested foods.

Digitalis   A drug that strengthens the force of contraction of the heart and slows the rate at which it beats. Digitalis drugs are used in the treatment of congestive heart failure and in the management of certain cardiac arrhythmias.

Dilatation   Enlargement of the blood vessels (usually arteries) or heart chambers.

Diuretic   A drug that increases the flow of urine and excretion of body fluid.

Dyspnea   Difficulty in breathing.

Echocardiography   A diagnostic technique that uses ultrasound waves to visualize and examine the heart structures. The pictorial record is called an echocardiogram.

Edema   Swelling of body tissue caused by a buildup of fluid.

Effusion   Accumulation of fluid between body tissues or in organs.

Ejection fraction   A measurement of left ventricular contraction that provides a useful measure of left ventricular function.

Electrocardiography   A diagnostic technique in which small electrodes are placed on the patient's chest, arms, and legs for the purpose of recording the electrical activity of the heart. The resulting tracing is called an electrocardiogram (EKG or ECG).

EKG   Electrocardiogram; a record of the electrical activity of the heart (sometimes called ECG).

Embolism   The blocking of a blood vessel by a clot (embolus) carried in the bloodstream from another location, where it was formed.

Embolus   A bit of matter (generally a blood clot) that drifts unattached in the bloodstream until it lodges in a blood vessel and frequently obstructs it.

Endocarditis   Infection of the inner lining of the heart chambers (endocardium).

Endothelium   The single layer of smooth, thin cells that lines the heart, blood vessels, lymph vessels, and body cavities.

Epinephrine   A hormone secreted by the adrenal gland upon stimulation of the sympathetic nervous system in response to stress such as anger or fear. It produces an increase in heart rate, blood pressure, cardiac output, and sugar metabolism.

EPS   Electrophysiological study. An invasive method for study of the basic electrical activity of the heart. Used in patients with serious arrhythmia.

Exercise echocardiogram   An echocardiographic study performed during and after exercise and correlated with a simultaneously performed electrocardiographic stress test. See *echocardiography*.

Exercise stress test   A test that symptomatically and electrocardiographically measures the heart's ability to tolerate an increased rate. See *stress test*.

Extrasystol   A premature beat, originating in either a ventricle or an atrium. See *ventricular premature beat*.

Fat   A component of most foods of plant or animal origin. An essential element in the diet.

Fatty acids   The basic chemical units of fats. These can be either saturated, monounsaturated, or polyunsaturated, depending on how many hydrogen atoms they hold. All dietary fats are a mixture of the three types of fatty acids in varying amounts.

Fiber   A nondigestible type of complex carbohydrate.

Fibrillation   Uncoordinated contraction of the heart muscle. It may involve the upper chambers (atrial fibrillation) or the lower chambers (ventricular fibrillation). See *ventricular fibrillation*.

Framingham Heart Study   An epidemiological heart study performed in a town in eastern Massachusetts since 1948, the source of well over four hundred scientific publications regarding the natural life histories and the specifics of all aspects of cardiovascular disease including risk factors, hypertension, and so forth.

HDL   See *high-density lipoproteins*.

Heart attack   See *myocardial infarction*.

Heart block   An arrhythmia caused by disruption (either partial or total) of the heart's electrical conduction pathways.

Heart failure   See *congestive heart failure*.

Heart-lung machine   A machine through which the bloodstream is diverted for pumping and oxygenation during heart surgery.

Heart murmur   An abnormal sound that can be heard through the chest with a stethoscope, resulting from turbulence in the bloodstream. It generally represents a malfunctioning heart valve.

Hemorrhage   Abnormal bleeding and loss of blood.

High blood pressure   See *hypertension*.

High-density lipoproteins (HDL)   Lipoproteins that contain a small amount of cholesterol and help to carry cholesterol away from body cells. The higher the HDL level, the better, as far as arteriosclerosis is concerned.

Holter monitor   A portable electrocardiograph worn by a patient over an extended period to assess the effects of activities of daily living on the heart rhythm and the electrocardiogram.

Hormone   Glandular secretion transported by the bloodstream to various organs in order to regulate vital functions and processes.

Hydrogenation   The chemical process that changes liquid vegetable oils (unsaturated fats) to a more solid (saturated) form.

Hypercholesterolemia   An excess of cholesterol in the blood.

Hypertension   High blood pressure. A condition characterized by excessive pressure within the arteries.

Hypertrophic cardiomyopathy   Enlargement of the left ventricle of the heart, resulting from a heart disease of unknown cause (possibly congenital). May cause congestive heart failure or sudden death.

Hypertrophy   Increased size and thickening of a muscle, causing strengthening of the force of contraction. It commonly occurs in the heart.

Hypotension   Low blood pressure.

Infarction   An irreversible injury to an area of the heart, usually as a result of a total blockage of the blood supply to the region. See *myocardial infarction*.

Insufficiency   See *regurgitation*.

Intravenous   Within a vein. A route for administration of drugs and other products.

Invasive procedure   A procedure that requires the entry of a needle, catheter, or other instrument into the body.

Ischemia   A local, usually temporary deficiency in oxygen supply to an organ or tissue due to obstruction or narrowing of the artery supplying that part. See also *silent myocardial ischemia*.

Ischemic heart disease   Heart disease most commonly resulting from atherosclerotic narrowing or obstruction of one or more of the coronary arteries.

Kidneys   The organs that regulate salt and water metabolism and remove waste products from the bloodstream to be excreted in the urine.

Lesion   An abnormal structural defect, such as the narrowing of a coronary artery, seen during surgery or on an angiogram.

LDL   See *low-density lipoproteins*.

Lipid   Fat or a fatlike substance; examples include cholesterol and tri-glycerides.

Lipoprotein   A blood compound consisting of lipid (fat) and protein molecules bound together. Lipoproteins carry fat and cholesterol through the bloodstream.

Low-density lipoproteins (LDL)   Lipoproteins that carry the largest amount of cholesterol in the blood. LDL is responsible for depositing cholesterol in the artery walls.

Lumen   The canal, duct, or cavity of a tubular organ.

Lungs   Two sponge-like organs that oxygenate the blood and expel gaseous waste (carbon dioxide) from the body.

Marfan syndrome   An inherited disease characterized by a generalized abnormality of the connective tissues of the body. It may have major effects on the heart, blood vessels, and skeletal and ocular systems.

Mediterranean diet   A diet inspired by the eating habits of the nations that border the Mediterranean Sea. The principal aspects of this diet include proportionally high consumption of olive oil, legumes, unrefined cereals, and fresh fruits and vegetables; moderate to high consumption of fish, seafood, and dairy products (mostly as cheese and yogurt); moderate wine consumption; and low consumption of nonfish meat products. A good deal of research accumulated over the last five decades indicates that the Mediterranean diet lowers the risk of heart disease. Some research shows that olive oil may be the main health-promoting part of the diet.

Milligram (mg)   A unit of weight equal to one-thousandth of a gram. There are 28,350 mg in one ounce.

Milligram/deciliter (mg/dl)   A method of expressing the concentration of solids in liquids. In blood cholesterol measurements, the weight of cholesterol (in milligrams) in a deciliter (about one-tenth of a quart) of blood.

Mitral valve   Heart valve through which blood passes from the left upper chamber (left atrium) to the main pumping chamber (left ventricle).

Mitral valve prolapse   A condition in which the mitral valve is improperly positioned and the edges of the valve leaflets do not come together properly.

Monounsaturated fats   Fats that lack a hydrogen band at one point in the carbon chain and tend to be associated with lower blood cholesterol content.

MRI   Magnetic resonance imaging; a non-X-ray method that can be used to study the heart and other organs.

Murmur   See *heart murmur.*

Myocardial infarction   An irreversible injury to an area of heart muscle caused by blockage of a coronary artery. See *infarction.*

Myocardial ischemia   Ischemia (see above) of the heart muscle.

Myocardium   The heart muscle.

Negative   In medicine, meaning normal or showing the absence of disease.

Niacin   B vitamin essential for cellular energy production; in large doses, a cholesterol-lowering agent.

Nicotine   A powerfully addictive drug that is the most dangerous component in tobacco cigarette smoke.

Nitrates   Drugs that relax the walls of blood vessels, especially arteries, causing them to dilate. Used mainly in the management of angina. See *nitroglycerine.*

Nitroglycerine   A drug that relaxes the walls of blood vessels, causing them to dilate. Used primarily for the treatment of angina attacks.

Noninvasive procedure   A medical procedure or test that does not require entry of a needle, catheter, or instrument into the body.

Nuclear cardiology   The area of cardiology that uses radioactive substances in heart studies.

Obesity   An excess of body fat. Should be distinguished from heaviness (body weight). Generally defined as at least 10 to 20 percent excess over "ideal" body weight based on one's age, height, and bone structure.

Occlusion   Total closure of a blood vessel.

Open-heart surgery   Surgery performed on the heart, its chambers, and/or the coronary arteries while the patient's blood is diverted through a heart-lung machine.

Orthopnea   A condition in which one has difficulty breathing except when sitting or standing upright.

Outpatient procedure   A test or procedure performed outside a hospital.

Oxygen   A gas that is essential for life and necessary for energy-producing chemical reactions in the cells of the body. Extracted from air inhaled into the lungs, it enters the bloodstream and is carried by the blood to the body tissues.

Pacemaker   A natural mechanism that generates tiny electrical impulses, setting the pace for the heartbeat. Artificial pacemakers are electronic devices that can be implanted under the skin and act as a substitute for a defective natural pacemaker. See *sinoatrial node*.

Palpitations   An awareness of the heartbeat. Often described as skipped, fluttering, forceful, and/or irregular heart activity.

Pericarditis   Inflammation of the pericardium (see below).

Pericardium   A thin membrane sac that surrounds the heart.

PET test   Positron-emission tomography. A heart test using special radionuclides.

Physiology   The science that studies the functions of body organs.

Plaque   Abnormal buildup of fatty deposits on the inner layer of an artery. Plaques reduce the internal diameter of the artery and may lead to total blockage. See *atheroma*.

Platelet   Tiny cell of the blood that plays an important part in the blood-clotting mechanism.

Platelet inhibitors   Drugs that inhibit blood-clot formation. Common examples are aspirin and Persantine.

Polyunsaturated fats   Fats so constituted chemically that they are capable of absorbing additional atoms of hydrogen. They are predominantly vegetable in origin, contain no cholesterol, and are usually liquid at room temperature.

Positive   In medicine, meaning abnormal or showing the presence of disease.

Potassium   An essential mineral that is necessary for muscle contraction.

Prognosis   Prediction or forecast of the probable course of a disease.

Prophylaxis   Prevention of disease. For example, in cardiology, the use of antibiotics to prevent an infection of the heart valves.

Protein   One of the three nutrients that supply calories to the body.

PTCA   Percutaneous transluminal coronary angioplasty. See *angioplasty*.

Pulmonary   Pertaining to the lungs.

Pulmonary artery   The large artery that transports unoxygenated blood from the right ventricle to the lungs. This is the only artery in the body that carries unoxygenated blood.

Pulmonary circulation   The circulation that carries unoxygenated blood from the heart to the lungs. It includes the right heart chambers, the main pulmonary artery, and the smaller pulmonary arteries.

Pulmonary edema   A severe form of congestive heart failure in which flooding of fluids into the air sacs in the lungs occurs, producing severe shortness of breath.

Pulmonary embolism   A condition in which a blood clot (embolus) has become dislodged, travels through the bloodstream, and becomes lodged in one of the arteries in the lungs.

Pulmonic valve   Heart valve through which unoxygenated blood passes from the right ventricle into the pulmonary artery and is then transported to the lungs.

Pulse   The expansion and contraction of an artery, which may be felt with the fingers.

QRS complex   Part of an electrocardiographic tracing.

Radioisotope   A radioactive material used in medical testing as well as in physical and biological research. Examples are thallium-201 and technetium-99m.

Radionuclide   A radioactive material. See *radioisotope*.

Rales   Moist crackling sounds that can be heard over the lower portion of the lungs, virtually always present in patients with congestive heart failure.

Regurgitation   In cardiology, the backward leakage of blood through a defective valve.

Renal   Pertaining to the kidneys.

Respiration   The act of breathing; the inhalation and exhalation of air.

Resuscitation   Restoration of breathing and heartbeat.

Revascularization   Improvement of the blood circulation, surgically or by other means.

Risk factor   A genetic or lifestyle habit, trait, condition, illness, or physical finding associated with increased risk or likelihood of a disease, such as coronary artery heart disease.

Saturated fats   Fats so constituted chemically that they are not capable of absorbing additional atoms of hydrogen. They are predominantly of animal origin (meat, dairy) and are usually solid at room temperature.

Septum   A dividing wall between two chambers. The ventricular septum is located between the two ventricles; the atrial septum is located between the two atria.

Serum   The clear, pale-yellow liquid that separates from the clot after blood coagulates. The liquid portion of blood that carries nutrients and other substances to and from the tissues.

Shock   A condition resulting from inadequate circulation. It may be due to loss of blood or to extreme weakness of the heart as a pump. Shock is marked by low blood pressure, rapid pulse, paleness, and cold, clammy skin.

Shunt   Diversion of blood between the two sides of the heart owing to the presence of an abnormal opening within or near the heart. Shunts may also occur between two vessels distant from the heart.

Silent heart disease   Symptom-free heart disorders, including ischemia, heart attacks, and even sudden death. See *silent myocardial ischemia.*

Silent myocardial ischemia   Symptom-free ischemia or inadequate coronary artery blood flow. See *silent heart disease.*

Sinoatrial node   The natural pacemaker of the heart. A small bundle of specialized cells that generates tiny electrical impulses that spread from the upper to the lower heart chambers, setting the pace of the heartbeat.

Sinus rhythm   Normal heart rhythm that occurs because of the electrical impulses initiated in the sinoatrial node.

Sodium   An essential mineral that is necessary to keep fluids distributed in the body. Table salt (sodium chloride) is nearly half sodium.

Spasm   Temporary contraction of a muscular segment. Occurs in arterial walls, usually making the lumen smaller. See *vasoconstriction* and *vasospasm.*

Sphygmomanometer   An instrument used to measure blood pressure.

Stenosis   Narrowing or stricture of an opening, blood vessel, or valve.

Stethoscope   A listening instrument that amplifies sounds coming from within the body.

Stress test   A test of cardiovascular health conducted by recording heart rate, blood pressure, electrocardiogram, and other measurements while a person undergoes physical exertion or drug-induced stress. See *exercise stress test.*

Stroke　Damage to the brain caused by an interruption of the blood flow to the brain.

Sudden cardiac death　Totally unexpected death occurring within one hour of the onset of symptoms in a victim with or without known preexisting heart disease.

Syncope　A fainting spell. A sudden loss of consciousness owing to a temporary reduction of blood flow and oxygen supply to the brain.

Systemic circulation　General circulation, as opposed to pulmonary circulation. It carries oxygenated blood to the entire body.

Systole　The period of each heartbeat during which the pumping chambers contract and eject their blood content. The systolic reading obtained in blood pressure measurement is the first, higher number.

Systolic blood pressure　The maximum arterial blood pressure, which occurs at the end of the left ventricle's contraction.

Tachycardia　An abnormally fast heart rate. Generally, anything over one hundred beats per minute is considered tachycardia.

Thallium stress test　A stress test conducted by injecting a small amount of radioactive substance (thallium) into the bloodstream and measuring its passage through the heart. See *stress test.*

Thrombolysis　Lysis (or dissolution) of a clot or thrombus, usually by drugs known as thrombolytic agents. See *TPA.*

Thrombosis　The formation of a blood clot (thrombus) that partially or completely blocks a blood vessel.

Total fat　The sum of saturated, monounsaturated, and polyunsaturated fats present in the diet.

TPA (tissue plasminogen activator)　A clot-dissolving enzyme occurring naturally in small amounts in the blood but now produced in large amounts by genetic engineering techniques.

Treadmill test　A stress test performed by using a motorized treadmill to produce physical stress. See *stress test.*

Tricuspid valve　Heart valve through which blood passes from the right atrium to the right ventricle.

Triglyceride　A common type of lipid (fat) carried in the bloodstream and found in fatty tissue, primarily ingested with fat in the diet.

Unsaturated fats　See *monounsaturated fats* and *polyunsaturated fats.*

Valve A flexible structure that regulates the flow of blood within the heart. It allows the blood to circulate in only one direction and prevents it from backing up.

Vascular Pertaining to blood vessels.

Vascular disease An ailment of the blood vessels often caused by atherosclerosis. It may occur anywhere in the body (brain, legs, coronary arteries, etc.).

Vasoconstriction Narrowing of blood vessels produced by contraction of the muscles in their walls. See *vasospasm.*

Vasodilator A drug that lowers blood pressure by relaxing the muscular walls of arteries, causing them to dilate.

Vasospasm Constriction or narrowing of an artery, leading to a decrease in its diameter and in the amount of blood it can deliver. See *vasoconstriction.*

Vein Any of the blood vessels that carry unoxygenated blood from all parts of the body back to the heart.

Ventricle One of the two pumping lower chambers of the heart. The left ventricle pumps oxygenated blood through the arteries to all parts of the body except the lungs. The right ventricle pumps unoxygenated blood through the pulmonary artery to the lungs.

Ventricular contraction Contraction of the left and right ventricles, the major chambers of the heart.

Ventricular fibrillation A heart arrhythmia characterized by rapid, chaotic electrical impulses, resulting in ineffectual contraction of the ventricles and loss of pulse and blood pressure. If it continues, death ensues.

Ventricular premature beats Premature beats or contractions originating in a ventricle.

Ventricular relaxation The phase of the heart cycle in which the ventricles are relaxed and fill with blood.

Ventriculogram An X-ray or radionuclide picture of the major chambers of the heart.

Very low-density lipoproteins Lipoproteins that transport cholesterol and triglycerides in the bloodstream.

BIBLIOGRAPHY

Ades P, Keteyian S, Wright J, et al. Increasing cardiac rehabilitation participation from 20% to 70%: a road map from the Million Hearts Cardiac Rehabilitation Collaborative Cdc-pdf [PDF-423K]. *Mayo Clin Proc.* 2016 November; doi: 10.1016/j.mayocp.2016.10.014.

Aguilar D, Goldhaber SZ, Gans DJ, et al.; Collaborative Study Group. Clinically unrecognized Q-wave myocardial infarction in patients with diabetes mellitus, systemic hypertension, and nephropathy. *Am J Cardiol.* 2004;94:337–339. doi: 10.1016/j.amjcard.2004.04.028.

American Psychiatric Association (APA). Diagnosis and Statistical Manual of Medical Disorders. 4th ed. Washington, DC: APA, 1994.

Ammar KA, Samee S, Makwana R, et al. Echocardiographic characteristics of electrocardiographically unrecognized myocardial infarctions in a community population. *Am J Cardiol.* 2005;96:1069–1075. doi: 10.1016/j.amjcard.2005.06.036.

Angell SY, Levings JL, Neiman A, Asma S, Merritt R. How policymakers can advance cardiovascular health. *Scientific American.* 2014 June:24–29.

ARIC Investigators. The Atherosclerosis Risk in Communities (ARIC) Study: design and objectives. *Am J Epidemiol.* 1989;129:687–702.

ARIC Investigators. *Manual 3: Surveillance Component Procedures Manual of Operations.* Version 6.4 (2015). Collaborative Studies Coordinating Center.

Asch FM, Shah S, Rattin C, et al. Lack of sensitivity of the electrocardiogram for detection of old myocardial infarction: a cardiac magnetic resonance imaging study. *Am Heart J.* 2006;152:742–748. doi: 10.1016/j.ahj.2006.02.037.

Auer PL, Stitziel NO. Genetic association studies in cardiovascular diseases: Do we have enough power? *Trends Cardiovasc Med.* 2017;27:397–404. doi: 10.1016/j.tcm.2017.03.005.

Benjamin EJ, Virani SS, Callaway CW, et al. Heart disease and stroke statistics—2018 update: a report from the American Heart Association. *Circulation.* 2018;137:e67–e92. doi: 10.1161/CIR.0000000000000558.

Bergelt C, Prescott E, Grønbaek M, Koch U, Johansen C. Stressful life events and cancer risk. *Brit J Cancer.* 2006;95:1579–81. doi: 10.1038/ sj.bjc.6603471.

Boland A, Gérardy J, Mossay D, Delapierre D, Seutin V. Pirlindole and dehydropirlindole protect rat cultured neuronal cells against oxidative stress-induced cell death through a mechanism unrelated to MAO-A inhibition. *Brit J Pharmacol.* 2002;135:713–720. doi: 10.1038/ sj.bjp.0704519.

Boland LL, Folsom AR, Sorlie PD, et al. Occurrence of unrecognized myocardial infarction in subjects aged 45 to 65 years (the ARIC study). *Am J Cardiol.* 2002;90:927–931.

Boscarino JA. A prospective study of PTSD and early-age heart disease mortality among Vietnam veterans: implications for surveillance and prevention. *Psychosom Med.* 2008;70:668–676. doi: 10.1097/PSY.0b013e31817bccaf.

Burg MM, Brandt C, Buta E, et al. Risk for incident hypertension associated with posttraumatic stress disorder in military veterans and the effect of posttraumatic stress disorder treatment. *Psychosom Med.* 2017;79:181–188.

Burgess DC, Hunt D, Li L, et al. Incidence and predictors of silent myocardial infarction in type 2 diabetes and the effect of fenofibrate: an analysis from the Fenofibrate Intervention and Event Lowering in Diabetes (FIELD) study. *Eur Heart J.* 2010;31:92–99. doi: 10.1093/eurheartj/ehp377.

Casper M, Kramer M, Quick H, Schieb L, Vaughan A, Greer S. Changes in the geographic patterns of heart disease mortality in the United States, 1973–2010. *Circulation.* 2016; 133:1171–1180 doi: 10.1161/CIRCULA TIONAHA.115.018663.

Charlson ME, Pompei P, Ales KL, MacKenzie CR. A new method of classifying prognostic comorbidity in longitudinal studies: development and validation. *J Chronic Dis.* 1987;40:373–383. doi: 10.1016/0021-9681(87)90171-8.

Chatterjee S, Biondi-Zoccai G, Abbate A, et al. Benefits of beta blockers in patients with heart failure and reduced ejection fraction: network meta-analysis. *BMJ.* 2013;346:f55. doi: 10.1136/bmj.f55.

Chatterjee S, Moeller C, Shah N, et al. Eplerenone is not superior to older and less expensive aldosterone antagonists. *Am J Med.* 2012;125:817–825. doi: 10.1016/j.amjmed.2011.12.018.

Cohen S, Janicki-Deverts D, Doyle WJ, et al. Chronic stress, glucocorticoid receptor resistance, inflammation, and disease risk. *P Natl Acad Sci USA.* 2012;109:5995–5999. doi: 10.1073/pnas.1118355109.

Cohen S, Tyrrell DA, Smith AP. Psychological stress and susceptibility to the common cold. *N Engl J Med.* 1991;325:606–612. doi: 10.1056 / NEJM199108293250903.

Connelly KA, MacIsaac AI, Jelinek VM. Stress, myocardial infarction, and the "tako-tsubo" phenomenon. *Heart.* 2004;90:e52. doi: 10.1136/hrt.2004.038851.

Crow RS, Prineas RJ, Hannan PJ, Grandits G, Blackburn H. Prognostic associations of Minnesota Code serial electrocardiographic change classification with coronary heart disease mortality in the Multiple Risk Factor Intervention Trial. *Am J Cardiol.* 1997;80:138–144.

D'Onofrio BM, Lahey BB, Turkheimer E, Lichtenstein P. Critical need for family-based, quasi-experimental designs in integrating genetic and social science research. *Am J Public Health.* 2013;103(Suppl 1):S46–S55. doi: 10.2105/AJPH.2013.301252.

Davis TM, Fortun P, Mulder J, Davis WA, Bruce DG; Fremantle Diabetes Study. Silent myocardial infarction and its prognosis in a community-based cohort of type 2 diabetic patients: the Fremantle Diabetes Study. *Diabetologia.* 2004;47:395–399. doi: 10.1007/s00125-004-1344-4.

de Torbal A, et al. Incidence of recognized and unrecognized myocardial infarction in men and women aged 55 and older: the Rotterdam study. *Eur Heart J.* 2006;27:729–736. doi: 10.1093/eurheartj/ehi707.

de Vries GJ, Olff M. The lifetime prevalence of traumatic events and posttraumatic stress disorder in the Netherlands. *J Trauma Stress.* 2009;22:259–267. doi: 10.1002/jts.20429.

Dunlay SM, Weston SA, Jacobsen SJ, et al. Risk factors for heart failure: a population-based case-control study. *Am J Med.* 2009;122:1023–1028. doi: 10.1016/j.amjmed.2009.04.022.

Engdahl J, Holmberg M, Karlson BW, Luepker R, Herlitz J. The epidemiology of out-of-hospital "sudden" cardiac arrest. *Resuscitation.* 2002;52:235–245. doi: 10.1016/S0300-9572(01)00464-6.

Fall K, Fang F, Mucci LA, et al. Immediate risk for cardiovascular events and suicide following a prostate cancer diagnosis: prospective cohort study. *PLoS Med.* 2009;6:e1000197. doi: 10.1371/journal.pmed.1000197.

Freeman AP, Giles RW, Walsh WF, et al. Regional left ventricular wall motion assessment: comparison of two-dimensional echocardiography and radionuclide angiography with contrast angiography in healed myocardial infarction. *Am J Cardiol.* 1985;56:8–12. doi: 10.1016/0002-9149(85)90556-9.

Frongillo E. Evaluating statistical interactions. https://www.cscu.cornell.edu/news/statnews/stnews64.pdf. Accessed July 29, 2015.

Ganesh SK, Arnett DK, Assimes TL, et al. Genetics and genomics for the prevention and treatment of cardiovascular disease: update: a scientific statement from the American Heart Association. *Circulation.* 2013 Dec;128:2813–2851.

220   *Bibliography*

Gilboa SM, Lee KA, Cogswell ME, et al. The National Birth Defects Prevention Study. *Birth Defects Res A Clin Mol Teratol.* 2014 Sep;100(9):647–657.

Gillespie CD, Wigington C, Hong Y; Centers for Disease Control and Prevention. Coronary heart disease and stroke deaths—United States, 2009. *MMWR.* 2013 Nov;62(03)(Suppl):157–160.

Go AS, Mozaffarian D, Roger VL, et al. Heart disease and stroke statistics—2014 update: a report from the American Heart Association. *Circulation.* 2014 Dec;129:e28–e292.

Gradus JL, Antonsen S, Svensson E, Lash TL, Resick PA, Hansen JG. Trauma, comorbidity, and mortality following diagnoses of severe stress and adjustment disorders: a nationwide cohort study. *Am J Epidemiol.* 2015;182:451–458. doi: 10.1093/aje/kwv066.

Gradus JL, Farkas DK, Svensson E, et al. Associations between stress disorders and cardiovascular disease events in the Danish population. *BMJ Open.* 2015;5:e009334. doi: 10.1136/bmjopen-2015-009334.

Gradus JL, Farkas DK, Svensson E, et al. Posttraumatic stress disorder and cancer risk: a nationwide cohort study. *Eur J Epidemiol.* 2015;30:563–568. doi: 10.1007/s10654-015-0032-7.

Greenwood JP, Maredia N, Younger JF, et al. Cardiovascular magnetic resonance and single-photon emission computed tomography for diagnosis of coronary heart disease (CE-MARC): a prospective trial. *Lancet.* 2012;379:453–460. doi: 10.1016/S0140-6736(11)61335-4.

Greer S, Kramer MR, Cook-Smith JN, Casper ML. Metropolitan racial residential segregation and cardiovascular mortality: exploring pathways. *J Urban Health.* 2014 Oct;91(3):499–509.

Greer S, Schieb L, Ritchey M, George M, Casper M. County health factors associated with avoidable deaths from cardiovascular disease in the United States, 2006–2010 [PDF-3M]. *Public Health Rep.* 2016 May–June;131:438–448.

Grimm RH Jr, Tillinghast S, Daniels K, et al. Unrecognized myocardial infarction: experience in the Multiple Risk Factor Intervention Trial (MRFIT). *Circulation.* 1987;75(pt 2):II6–II8.

Gros DF, Price M, Magruder KM, Frueh BC. Symptom overlap in posttraumatic stress disorder and major depression. *Psychiatry Res.* 2012;196:267–270. doi: 10.1016/j.psychres.2011.10.022.

Gussak I, Wright RS, Bjerregaard P, et al. False-negative and false-positive ECG diagnoses of Q wave myocardial infarction in the presence of right bundle-branch block. *Cardiology.* 2000;94:165–172. doi: 10.1159/000047312.

Harvey AG, Bryant RA. The relationship between acute stress disorder and posttraumatic stress disorder: a 2-year prospective evaluation. *J Consult Clin Psychol.* 1999;67:985–988. doi: 10.1037/0022-006X.67.6.985.

Heidenreich PA, Albert NM, Allen LA, et al. Forecasting the impact of heart failure in the United States: a policy statement from the American Heart Association. *Circ Heart Fail.* 2013;6:606–619. doi: 10.1161/HHF.0b013e318291329a [PMC free article].

Huffman MD, Berry JD, Ning H, et al. Lifetime risk for heart failure among white and black Americans: cardiovascular lifetime risk pooling project. *J Am Coll Cardiol.* 2013;61:1510–1517. doi: 10.1016/j.jacc.2013.01.022.

Hulley S, Grady D, Bush T, et al. Randomized trial of estrogen plus progestin for secondary prevention of coronary heart disease in postmenopausal women: Heart and Estrogen/Progestin Replacement Study (HERS) Research Group. *JAMA.* 1998;280:605–613.

Jónsdóttir LS, Sigfusson N, Sigvaldason H, Thorgeirsson G. Incidence and prevalence of recognised and unrecognised myocardial infarction in women: the Reykjavik study. *Eur Heart J.* 1998;19:1011–1018.

Jordan HT, Miller-Archie SA, Cone JE, Morabia A, Stellman SD. Heart disease among adults exposed to the September 11, 2001 World Trade Center disaster: results from the World Trade Center Health Registry. *Prev Med.* 2011;53:370–376. doi: 10.1016/j.ypmed.2011.10.014.

Jordan HT, Stellman SD, Morabia A, et al. Cardiovascular disease hospitalizations in relation to exposure to the September 11, 2001 World Trade Center disaster and posttraumatic stress disorder. *J Am Heart Assoc.* 2013;2:e000431. doi: 10.1161/JAHA.113.000431.

Kannel WB. Prevalence and clinical aspects of unrecognized myocardial infarction and sudden unexpected death. *Circulation.* 1987;75:II4–II5.

Kannel WB, Abbott RD. Incidence and prognosis of unrecognized myocardial infarction: an update on the Framingham study. *N Engl J Med.* 1984;311:1144–1147. doi: 10.1056/NEJM198411013111802.

Kannel WB, Cupples LA, Gagnon DR. Incidence, precursors and prognosis of unrecognized myocardial infarction. *Adv Cardiol.* 1990;37:202–214.

Kannel WB, McNamara PM, Feinleib M, Dawber TR. The unrecognized myocardial infarction: fourteen-year follow-up experience in the Framingham study. *Geriatrics.* 1970 Jan;25(1):75–87.

Kannel WB, Sorlie P, McNamara PM. Prognosis after initial myocardial infarction: the Framingham study. *Am J Cardiol.* 1979;44:53–59.

Kehl DW, Farzaneh-Far R, Na B, Whooley MA. Prognostic value of electrocardiographic detection of unrecognized myocardial infarction in persons with stable coronary artery disease: data from the Heart and Soul Study. *Clin Res Cardiol.* 2011;100:359–366. doi: 10.1007/s00392-010-0255-2.

Kessler RC, Aguilar-Gaxiola S, Alonso J, et al. Trauma and PTSD in the WHO World Mental Health Surveys. *Eur J Psychotraumatol.* 2017;8(Suppl 5):1353383. doi: 10.1080/20008198.2017.1353383.

Khatibzadeh S, Farzadfar F, Oliver J, et al. Worldwide risk factors for heart failure: a systematic review and pooled analysis. *Int J Cardiol.* 2013;168:1186–1194. doi: 10.1016/j.ijcard.2012.11.065.

Khera AV, Emdin CA, Drake I, et al. Genetic risk, adherence to a healthy lifestyle, and coronary disease. *N Engl J Med.* 2016;375:2349–2358. doi: 10.1056/NEJMoa1605086.

Koenen KC, Sumner JA, Gilsanz P, et al. Post-traumatic stress disorder and cardiometabolic disease: improving causal inference to inform practice. *Psychol Med.* 2017;47:209–225. doi: 10.1017/S0033291716002294.

Kubzansky LD, Koenen KC, Jones C, Eaton WW. A prospective study of posttraumatic stress disorder symptoms and coronary heart disease in women. *Health Psychol.* 2009;28:125–130. doi: 10.1037/0278-6133.28.1.125.

Kubzansky LD, Koenen KC, Spiro A III, Vokonas PS, Sparrow D. Prospective study of posttraumatic stress disorder symptoms and coronary heart disease in the Normative Aging Study. *Arch Gen Psychiatry.* 2007;64:109–116. doi: 10.1001/archpsyc.64.1.109.

Kwong RY, Chan AK, Brown KA, et al. Impact of unrecognized myocardial scar detected by cardiac magnetic resonance imaging on event-free survival in patients presenting with signs or symptoms of coronary artery disease. *Circulation.* 2006;113:2733–2743. doi: 10.1161/CIRCULATIONAHA.105.570648.

Lambert PC, Royston P. Further development of flexible parametric models for survival analysis. *Stata J.* 2009;9:265–290. doi: 10.1177/1536867X0900900206.

Law MR, Watt HC, Wald NJ. The underlying risk of death after myocardial infarction in the absence of treatment. *Arch Intern Med.* 2002;162:2405–2410. doi: 10.1001/archinte.162.21.2405.

Li J, Precht DH, Mortensen PB, Olsen J. Mortality in parents after death of a child in Denmark: a nationwide follow-up study. *Lancet.* 2003;361:363–367. doi: 10.1016/S0140-6736(03)12387-2.

Ludvigsson JF, Otterblad-Olausson P, Pettersson BU, Ekbom A. The Swedish personal identity number: possibilities and pitfalls in healthcare and medical research. *Eur J Epidemiol.* 2009;24:659–667. doi: 10.1007/s10654-009-9350-y.

Margolis JR, Kannel WS, Feinleib M, Dawber TR, McNamara PM. Clinical features of unrecognized myocardial infarction—silent and symptomatic. Eighteen year follow-up: the Framingham study. *Am J Cardiol.* 1973;32:1–7.

Medalie JH, Goldbourt U. Unrecognized myocardial infarction: five-year incidence, mortality, and risk factors. *Ann Intern Med.* 1976;84:526–531.

Nadelmann J, Frishman WH, Ooi WL, et al. Prevalence, incidence and prognosis of recognized and unrecognized myocardial infarction in persons aged 75 years or older: the Bronx Aging Study. *Am J Cardiol.* 1990;66:533–537.

Mirambeau AM, Wang G, Ruggles L, Dunet DO. A cost analysis of a community health worker program in rural Vermont. *J Community Health.* 2013 Dec;38(6):1050–1057.

Moyer VA, U.S. Preventive Services Task Force screening for coronary heart disease with electrocardiography: U.S. Preventive Services Task Force recommendation statement. *Ann Intern Med.* 2012;157:512–518.

Mozaffarian D, Benjamin EJ, Go AS, et al.; American Heart Association Statistics Committee and Stroke Statistics Subcommittee. Heart disease and stroke statistics—2015 update: a report from the American Heart Association. *Circulation.* 2015;131:e29–e322. doi: 10.1161/CIR.0000000000000152.

National Collaborating Centre for Mental Health. *Post-traumatic Stress Disorder: The Management of PTSD in Adults and Children in Primary and Secondary Care.* Leicester, UK: Gaskell, 2005.

Nikolaou K, Knez A, Rist C, et al. Accuracy of 64-MDCT in the diagnosis of ischemic heart disease. *AJR Am J Roentgenol.* 2006;187:111–117. doi: 10.2214/AJR.05.1697.

Nkomo VT, Gardin JM, Skelton TN, et al. Burden of valvular heart diseases: a population-based study. *Lancet.* 2006;368:1005–1011. doi: 10.1016/S0140-6736(06)69208-8.

Norhammar A, Mellbin L, Cosentino F. Diabetes: prevalence, prognosis and management of a potent cardiovascular risk factor. *Eur J Prev Cardiol.* 2017;24(Suppl):52–60. doi: 10.1177/2047487317709554.

O'Donovan A, Cohen BE, Seal KH, et al. Elevated risk for autoimmune disorders in Iraq and Afghanistan veterans with posttraumatic stress disorder. *Biol Psychiatry.* 2015;77:365–374. doi: 10.1016/j.biopsych.2014.06.015.

Pride YB, Piccirillo BJ, Gibson CM. Prevalence, consequences, and implications for clinical trials of unrecognized myocardial infarction. *Am J Cardiol.* 2013;111:914–918. doi: 10.1016/j.amjcard.2012.11.042.

Prineas RJ, Crow RS, Blackburn H. *The Minnesota Code Manual of Electrocardiographic Findings.* Boston, MA: John Wright PSB, 1982.

Prineas RJ, Crow RS, Zhang ZM. *The Minnesota Code Manual of Electrocardiographic Findings.* 2nd ed. London: Springer: 2010.

Qureshi WT, Zhang ZM, Chang PP, et al. Silent myocardial infarction and long-term risk of heart failure: the ARIC Study. *J Am Coll Cardiol.* 2018;71:1–8. doi: 10.1016/j.jacc.2017.10.071.

Ritchey MD, Wall HK, Gillespie C, George MG, Jamal A. Million hearts: prevalence of leading cardiovascular disease risk factors—United States, 2005–2012. *MMWR.* 2014 May;63(21):462–467.

Rosamond WD, Chambless LE, Heiss G, et al. Twenty-two-year trends in incidence of myocardial infarction, coronary heart disease mortality, and case fatality in 4 US communities, 1987–2008. *Circulation.* 2012;125:1848–1857. doi: 10.1161/CIRCULATIONAHA.111.047480.

Rosengren A, Hawken S, Ounpuu S, et al.; INTERHEART Investigators. Association of psychosocial risk factors with risk of acute myocardial infarction in 11119 cases and 13648 controls from 52 countries (the INTERHEART study): case-control study. *Lancet.* 2004;364:953–962. doi: 10.1016/S0140 -6736(04)17019-0.

Rosenman RH, Friedman M, Jenkins CD, Straus R, Wurm M, Kositchek R. Clinically unrecognized myocardial infarction in the Western Collaborative Group Study. *Am J Cardiol.* 1967;19:776–782.

Roy SS, Foraker RE, Girton RA, Mansfield AJ. Posttraumatic stress disorder and incident heart failure among a community-based sample of US veterans. *Am J Public Health.* 2015;105:757–763. doi: 10.2105/AJPH.2014.302342.

Safford MM, Brown TM, Muntner PM, et al.; REGARDS Investigators. Association of race and sex with risk of incident acute coronary heart disease events. *JAMA.* 2012;308:1768–1774. doi: 10.1001/jama.2012.14306.

Scherrer JF, Salas J, Cohen BE, et al. Comorbid conditions explain the association between posttraumatic stress disorder and incident cardiovascular disease. *J Am Heart Assoc.* 2019;8:e011133. doi: 10.1161/JAHA.118.011133.

Sharkey SW, Lesser JR, Zenovich AG, et al. Acute and reversible cardiomyopathy provoked by stress in women from the United States. *Circulation.* 2005;111:472–479. doi: 10.1161/01.CIR.0000153801.51470.EB.

Sheifer SE, Gersh BJ, Yanez ND III, Ades PA, Burke GL, Manolio TA. Prevalence, predisposing factors, and prognosis of clinically unrecognized myocardial infarction in the elderly. *J Am Coll Cardiol.* 2000;35:119–126.

Sheifer SE, Manolio TA, Gersh BJ. Unrecognized myocardial infarction. *Ann Intern Med.* 2001;135:801–811.

Shen Q, Lu D, Schelin ME, et al. Injuries before and after diagnosis of cancer: nationwide register based study. *BMJ.* 2016;354:i4218. doi: 10.1136/bmj .i4218.

Shettigar UR, Pannuri A, Barbier GH, et al. Significance of anterior Q waves in left anterior fascicular block—a clinical and noninvasive assessment. *Clin Cardiol.* 2002;25:19–22. doi: 10.1002/clc.4950250106.

Shlipak MG, Elmouchi DA, Herrington DM, Lin F, Grady D, Hlatky MA; Heart and Estrogen/Progestin Replacement Study Research Group. The incidence of unrecognized myocardial infarction in women with coronary heart disease. *Ann Intern Med.* 2001;134:1043–1047.

Short V, Ivory-Walls T, Smith L, Loustalot F. The Mississippi Delta Cardiovascular Health Examination Survey (Delta CHES): study design and methods. *Epidemiology Research International.* 2014 Feb;Article ID 861461.

Sigurdsson E, Thorgeirsson G, Sigvaldason H, Sigfusson N. Unrecognized myocardial infarction: epidemiology, clinical characteristics, and the prognostic role of angina pectoris: the Reykjavik study. *Ann Intern Med.* 1995;122:96–102.

Song H, Fang F, Tomasson G, et al. Association of stress-related disorders with subsequent autoimmune disease. *JAMA.* 2018;319:2388–2400. doi: 10.1001/jama.2018.7028.

Steptoe A, Kivimäki M. Stress and cardiovascular disease. *Nat Rev Cardiol.* 2012;9:360–370. doi: 10.1038/nrcardio.2012.45.

Stokes J III, Dawber TR. The silent coronary: the frequency and clinical characteristics of unrecognized myocardial infarction in the Framingham study. *Ann Intern Med.* 1959;50:1359–1369.

Sumner JA, Kubzansky LD, Elkind MSV, et al. Trauma exposure and posttraumatic stress disorder symptoms predict onset of cardiovascular events in women. *Circulation.* 2015;132:251–259. doi: 10.1161/CIRCULATIONAHA.114.014492.

Sumner JA, Kubzansky LD, Kabrhel C, et al. Associations of trauma exposure and posttraumatic stress symptoms with venous thromboembolism over 22 years in women. *J Am Heart Assoc.* 2016;5:e003197. doi: 10.1161/JAHA.116.003197.

Thygesen K, Alpert JS, Jaffe AS, Simoons ML, Chaitman BR, White HD; Joint ESC/ACCF/AHA/WHF Task Force for the Universal Definition of Myocardial Infarction. Third universal definition of myocardial infarction. *Circulation.* 2012;126:2020–2035.

Thygesen K, Alpert JS, White HD; Joint ESC/ACCF/AHA/WHF Task Force for the Redefinition of Myocardial Infarction. Universal definition of myocardial infarction. *Circulation.* 2007;116:2634–2653.

Ursano RJ, Bell C, Eth S, et al.; Work Group on ASD and PTSD, Steering Committee on Practice Guidelines. Practice guideline for the treatment of patients with acute stress disorder and posttraumatic stress disorder. *Am J Psychiatry.* 2004;161(Suppl):3–31.

Vaccarino V, Goldberg J, Rooks C, et al. Post-traumatic stress disorder and incidence of coronary heart disease: a twin study. *J Am Coll Cardiol.* 2013;62:970–978. doi: 10.1016/j.jacc.2013.04.085.

Vaid I, Ahmed K, May D, Manheim D. The WISEWOMAN Program: smoking prevalence and key approaches to smoking cessation among participants, July 2008–June 2013. *Journal of Women's Health.* 2014 Feb;23(4):288–295.

Vaughan A, Quick H, Pathak EB, Kramer M, Casper M. Disparities in temporal and geographic patterns of declining heart disease mortality by race and sex in the United States, 1973–2010. *J Am Heart Assoc.* 2015 Dec;4(12):e002567, doi: 10.1161/JAHA.115.002567.

Veazie M, Ayala C, Schieb LJ, Dai S, Henderson JA, Cho P. Trends and disparities in heart disease mortality among American Indians/Alaska Natives, 1990–2009. *Am J Public Health.* 2014 April;104(S3):S359–S367. doi: 10.2105/AJPH.2013.301715.

Weir RA, McMurray JJ. Epidemiology of heart failure and left ventricular dysfunction after acute myocardial infarction. *Curr Heart Fail Rep.* 2006;3:175–180. doi: 10.1007/s11897-006-0019-5.

Wentworth BA, Stein MB, Redwine LS, et al. Post-traumatic stress disorder: a fast track to premature cardiovascular disease? *Cardiol Rev.* 2013;21:16–22. doi: 10.1097/CRD.0b013e318265343b.

White AD, Folsom AR, Chambless LE, Sharret AR, Yang K, Conwill D, et al. Community surveillance of coronary heart disease in the Atherosclerosis Risk in Communities (ARIC) Study: methods and initial two years' experience. *J Clin Epidemiol.* 1996;49:223–233.

Will J, Loustalot F, Hong Y. National trends in visits to physician offices and outpatient clinics for angina: 1995–2010. *Circ Cardiovasc Qual.* 2014 Jan;7(1):110–117. doi: 10.1161/CIRCOUTCOMES.113.000450.

Will JC, Yuan K, Ford ES. National trends in the prevalence and medical history of angina: 1988–2012. *Circ Cardiovasc Qual.* 2014 May;7(3):407–413. doi: 10.1161/CIRCOUTCOMES.113.000779.

World Health Organization. Cardiovascular diseases (CVDs). May 17, 2017. https://www.who.int/news-room/fact-sheets/detail/cardiovascular-diseases-(cvds). Accessed December 13, 2019.

World Health Organization. *The ICD-10 Classification of Mental and Behavioral Disorders: Clinical Description and Diagnostic Guidelines.* Geneva: WHO, 1992.

Wu E, Judd RM, Vargas JD, et al. Visualisation of presence, location, and transmural extent of healed Q-wave and non-Q-wave myocardial infarction. *Lancet.* 2001;357:21–28. doi: 10.1016/S0140-6736(00)03567-4.

Yancy CW, Jessup M, Bozkurt B, et al. 2017 ACC/AHA/HFSA focused update of the 2013 ACCF/AHA guideline for the management of heart failure: a report of the American College of Cardiology/American Heart Association Task Force on Clinical Practice Guidelines and the Heart Failure Society of America. *Circulation*. 2017;136:e137–e161. doi: 10.1161 /CIR.0000000000000509.

Yang Q, Yuan K, Gregg E, et al. Trends and clustering of cardiovascular health metrics among US adolescents 1988–2010. *J Adolesc Health*. 2014 Oct;55(4):513–520. doi: 10.1016/j.jadohealth.2014.03.013.

Yang Q, Zhang Z, Gregg EW, Flanders WD, Merritt R, Hu FB. Added sugar intake and cardiovascular diseases mortality among US adults. *JAMA Intern Med*. 2014 April;174(4):516–524.

Yano K, MacLean CJ. The incidence and prognosis of unrecognized myocardial infarction in the Honolulu, Hawaii, Heart Program. *Arch Intern Med*. 1989;149:1528–1532.

Ziegelstein RC. Acute emotional stress and cardiac arrhythmias. *JAMA*. 2007;298:324–329. doi: 10.1001/jama.298.3.324.

ACKNOWLEDGMENTS

A book of this nature requires many hands on deck.

First, I would like to give special thanks to my creative collaborator, Greg Ptacek, for captaining the book from proposal to final manuscript and navigating it through the ever-changing shoals of today's publishing world. I also am grateful to my editor, Suzanne I. Staszak-Silva, for initially believing in the project and then providing the book safe harbor at Rowman & Littlefield.

I wish to thank my former partners and fellow cardiologists, as well as the entire staff, at the Cardiology Medical Group of Southern California and my former academic colleagues at UCLA School of Medicine. Their professionalism and dedication to the profession of medicine always allowed me to do my job better.

Also, I wish express sincere gratitude to the thousands of patients whom I have treated as a doctor over the past seven decades. As this book illustrates, so much has changed in cardiology since I first began practicing medicine; however, the eternal bond between physician and patient remains constant. The dedication of my professional life to helping those in need has been a privilege.

And last but never least, I wish to express love and thanks for the support from my beautiful wife, Molinda, along with my son David, daughter Laura, and grandchildren Kai-Lilly, Huston, and Benny.

INDEX

AA. *See* Alcoholics Anonymous
AARP, 101
abdominal aortic aneurysm, 118
acebutolol (Sectral), 173
ACE inhibitors. *See* angiotensin converting enzyme inhibitors
adipokines, 113
adrenaline (epinephrine), 23, 130, 139
advanced cholesterol panel, 165
African Americans, 75–76, 145
age: in ASCVD, 98; atrial fibrillation and, 63; CHD and, 62–64; cocaine use by, 129; in DIY cardiac risk test, 194; heart attacks and, 59–60; hypertension and, 63, 73, 75; SMI and, 57–64, 149–50; of sudden cardiac death, 38–39; women and, 59–60
AHA. *See* American Heart Association
AI. *See* artificial intelligence
alcohol: benefits of, 125–26; binge drinking of, 124–25; CHD and, 120–22; deaths from, 121; per capital consumption of, 120–21; in pregnancy, 126; stress and, 135
Alcoholics Anonymous (AA), 125

Alcoholism: Clinical & Experimental Research, 121
Allogenic Heart Stem Cells to Achieve Myocardial Regeneration (ALLSTAR), 187
Altace. *See* ramipril
Alzheimer's disease, 1
amadhumeha (honey urine), 82
American College of Cardiology, 72, 166–67
American Diabetes Association, 84
American Heart Association (AHA), 72, 166–67; on diabetes, 80; on LDL, 84; on Mediterranean-style diet, 90, 91–92; on sedentary lifestyle, 95, 99
American Heart Journal, 183
American Journal of Cardiology, 97
American Medical Association, 90
American National Health and Nutrition Examination Survey, 123
amlodipine (Norvasc), 173
Ancestry.com, 54
angina. *See* chest pain
anginal equivalents, 41
angiotensin converting enzyme inhibitors (ACE inhibitors), 172

ABOUT THE AUTHOR

Dr. Harold L. Karpman received his bachelor's degree when he graduated from the University of California, San Francisco. He started his four-year medical school training, graduating and receiving his medical degree in June 1954. After extensive postgraduate training—his residencies were at the Los Angeles County General Hospital and Beth Israel Hospital at Harvard Medical School—he started his medical practice in cardiology in 1959.

Dr. Karpman was a clinical professor of medicine for the David Geffen School of Medicine, University of California, Los Angeles. He started his cardiology practice along with Drs. Daniel Bleifer and Selvyn Bleifer in 1960 (Cardiovascular Medical Group of Southern California) in Beverly Hills, California. He retired from his practice at the age of ninety-one in April 2018. He founded Cardio-Dynamics Laboratories, Inc., creator of the world's first Holter twenty-four-hour cardiac recording monitor. He also founded the Cardiovascular Research Foundation of Southern California—a nonprofit public entity dedicated to community-funded cardiovascular research, where he still serves on the board of directors. Dr. Karpman also served as chairman of the board of Western Cardiovascular Network, and he continues to serve on the board of governors of Cedars-Sinai Medical Center.

Aside from his successful career as a doctor, Dr. Karpman is a much sought after speaker, lecturer, and published author. He has written several books, including *Your Second Life* and *Preventing Silent Heart Disease*, both for lay people on heart disease, and more than one hundred peer-reviewed papers and presentations. He is an authority on the economics of health-care delivery and managed care and is a celebrated expert on all aspects of clinical and consultative cardiology. His curriculum vitae lists over 150 articles.

Dr. Karpman attributes his success to his education, mentors he had along the way, and his passion for helping his patients and their families. He says he found his work very gratifying and hopes that others will consider a career in cardiology.

When not working, he enjoys opera, classical music, tennis, Woody Allen movies, and time with his wife and family.

CPSIA information can be obtained
at www.ICGtesting.com
Printed in the USA
LVHW092026310821
696585LV00001B/28

9 781538 136553